Effective Prevention and Treatment of Substance Use Disorders for Racial and Ethnic Minorities

Edited by Erick Guerrero and Tenie Khachikian

Published in London, United Kingdom

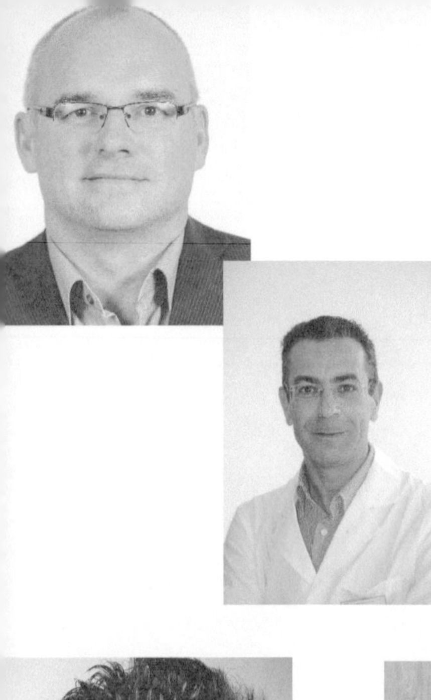
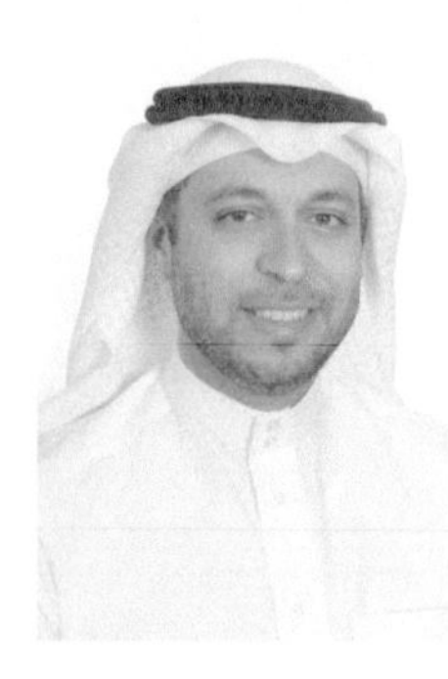
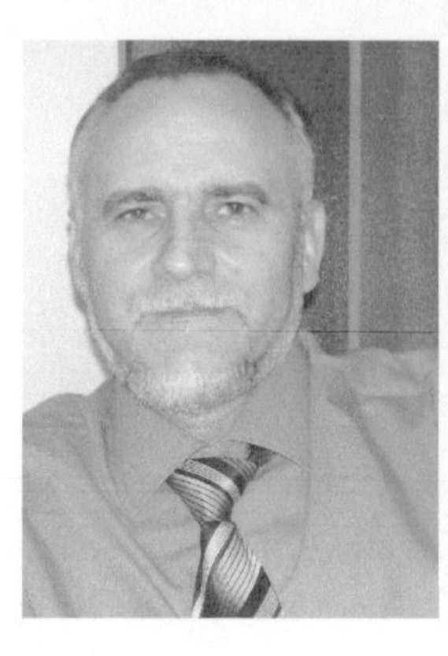
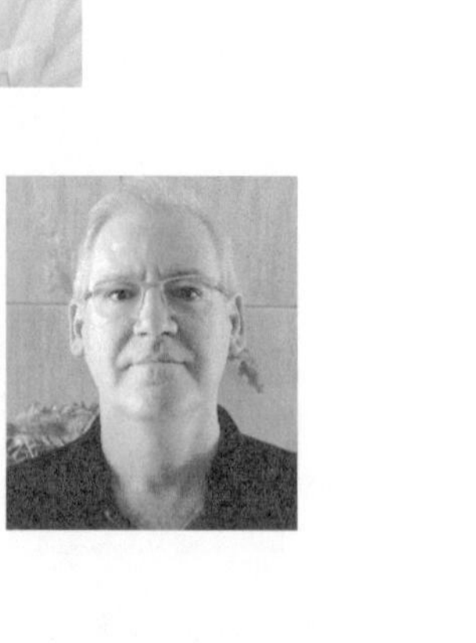
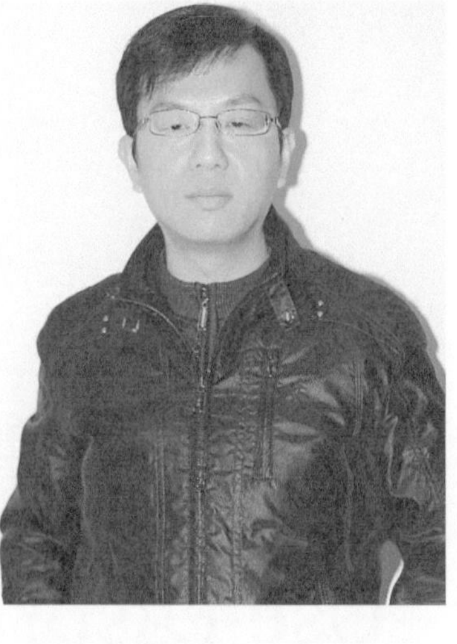

IntechOpen

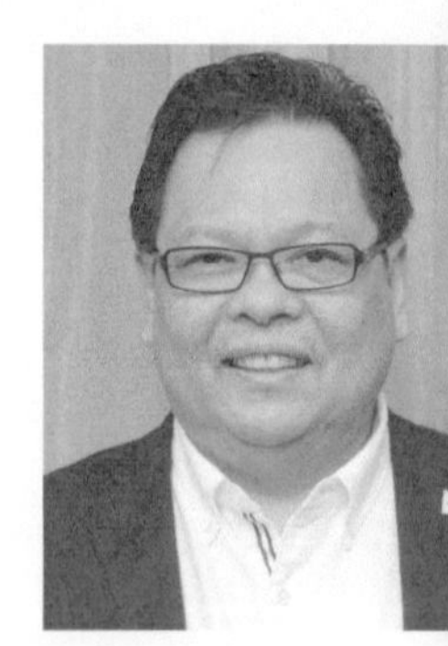
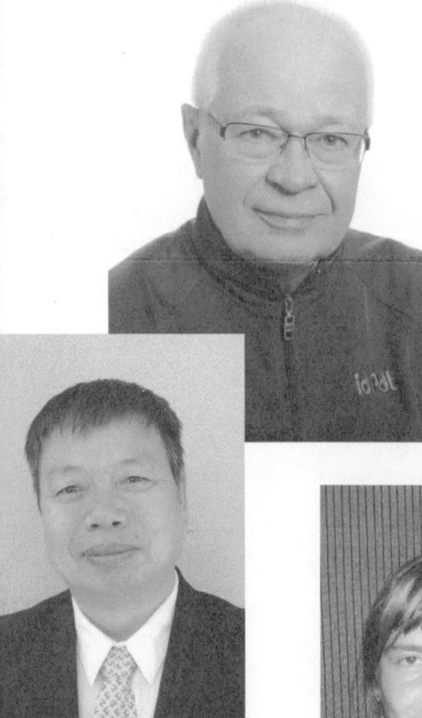
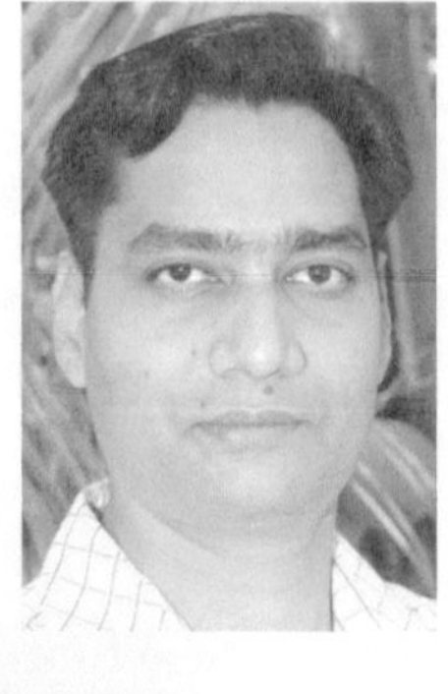
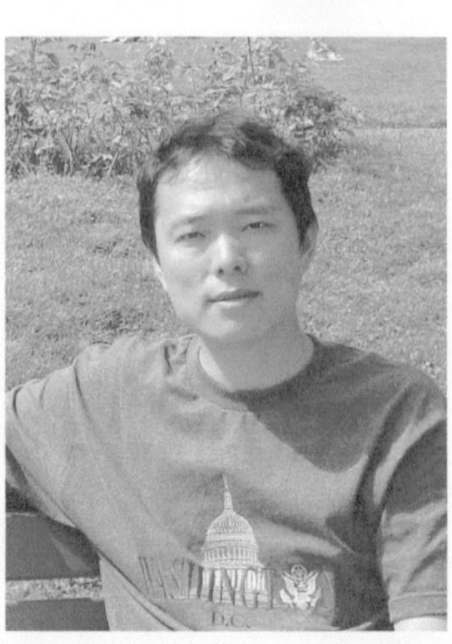
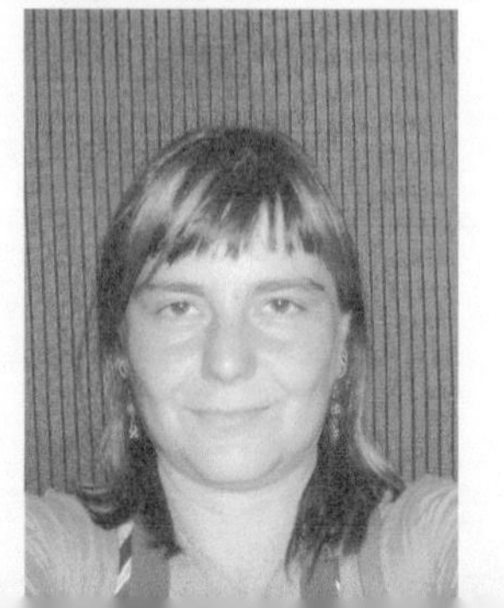

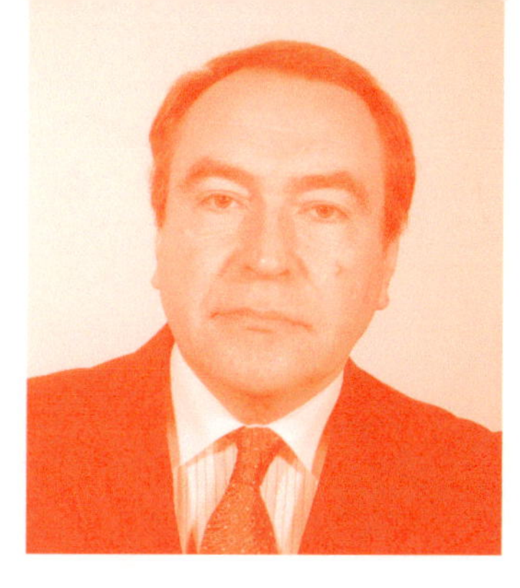
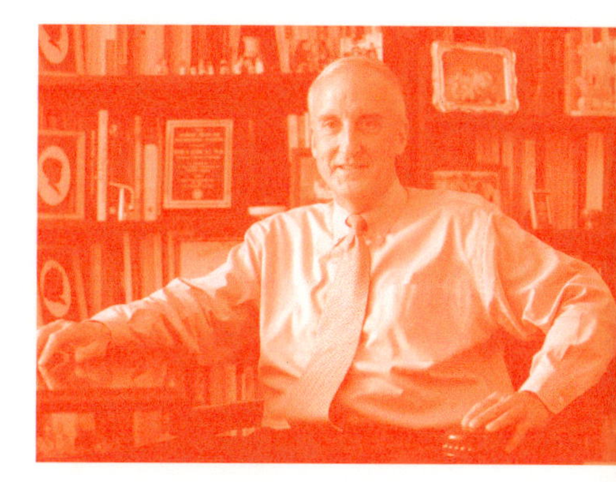
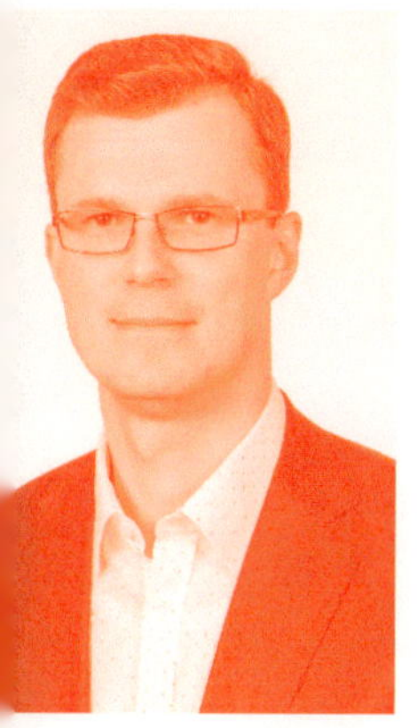
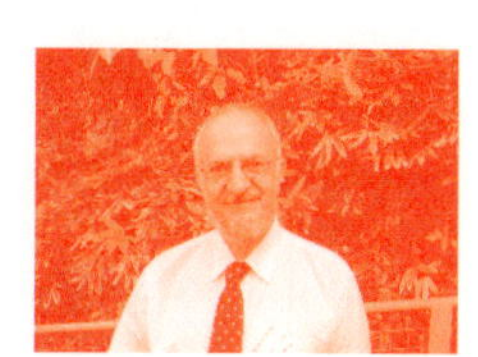
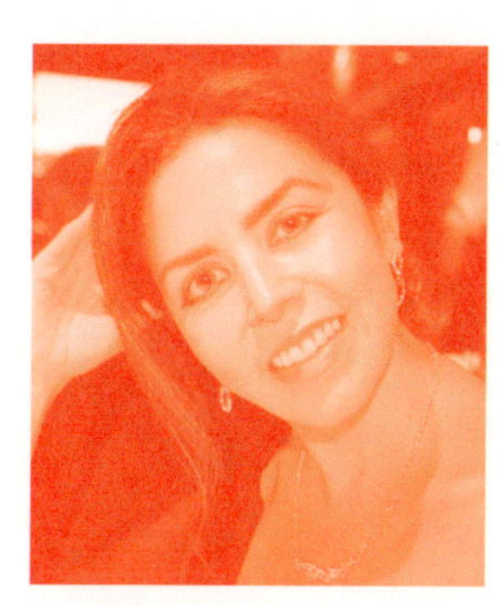

Supporting open minds since 2005

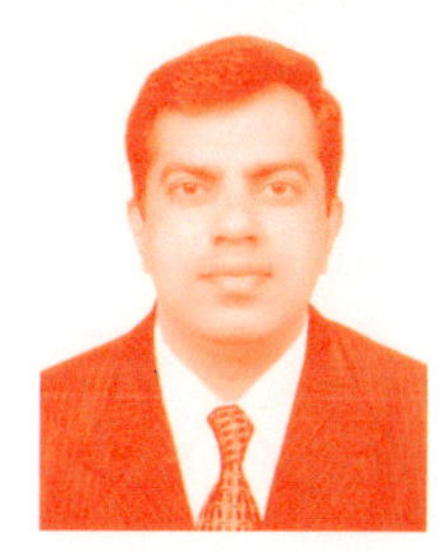
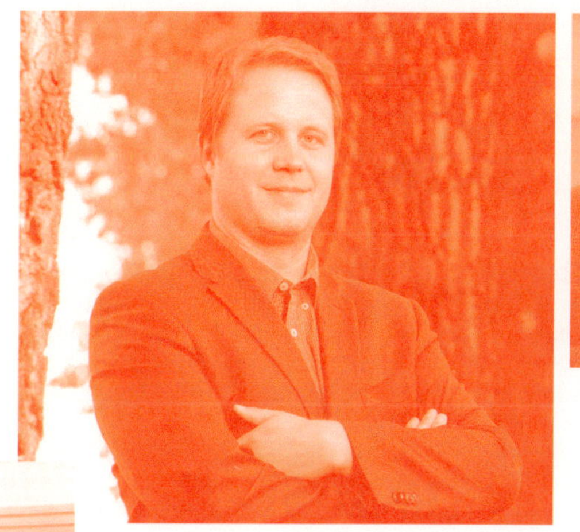
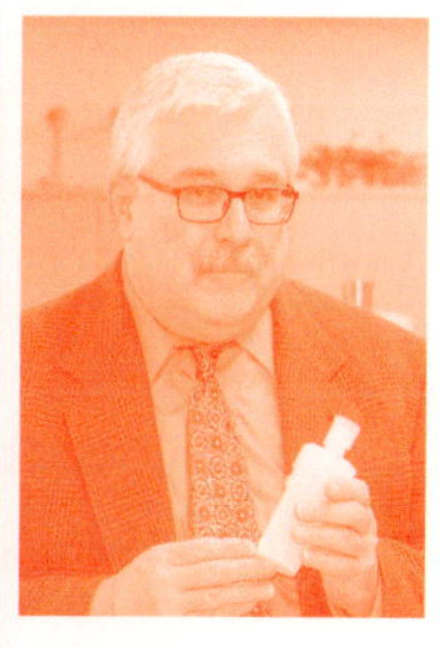
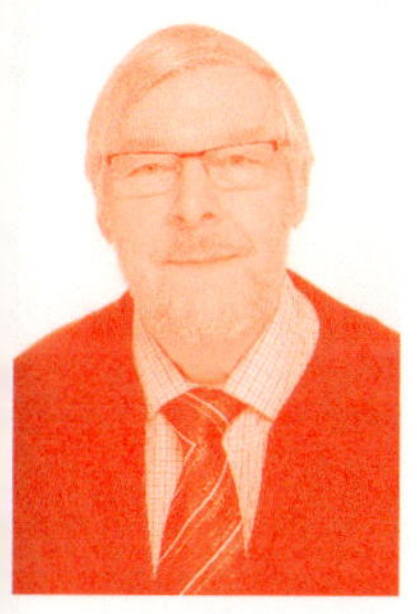
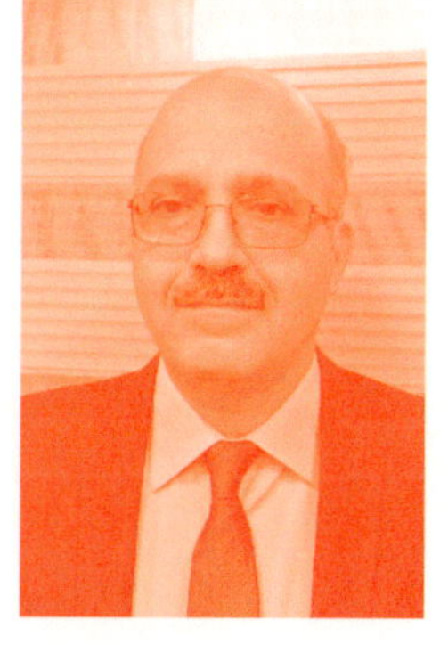
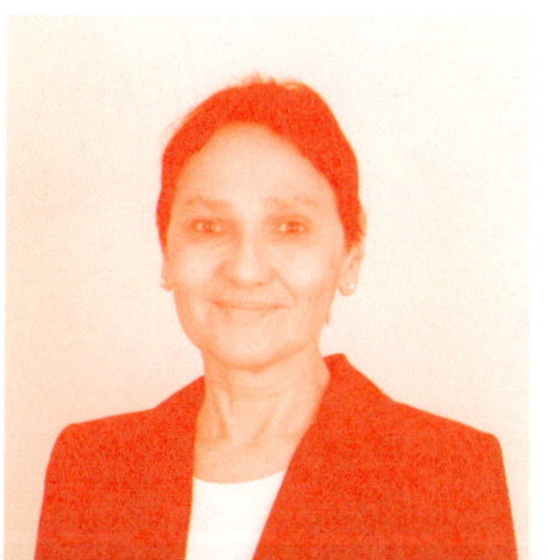
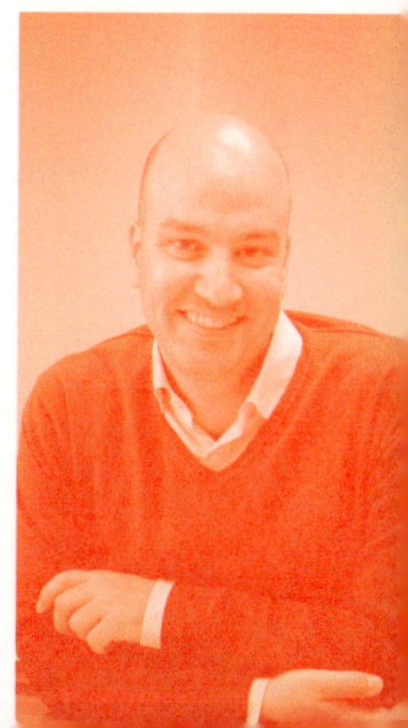

Effective Prevention and Treatment of Substance Use Disorders for Racial and Ethnic Minorities
http://dx.doi.org/10.5772/intechopen.78464
Edited by Erick Guerrero and Tenie Khachikian

Contributors
Erick Guerrero, Tenie Khachikian, Jemima A. Frimpong, Daniel L. Howard, Shernaaz Carelse, Richard Cervantes, Elias Koutantos

First published in London, United Kingdom, 2020 by IntechOpen
IntechOpen is the global imprint of INTECHOPEN LIMITED, registered in England and Wales, registration number: 11086078, 7th floor, 10 Lower Thames Street, London, EC3R 6AF, United Kingdom
Printed in Croatia

British Library Cataloguing-in-Publication Data
A catalogue record for this book is available from the British Library

Additional hard and PDF copies can be obtained from orders@intechopen.com

Effective Prevention and Treatment of Substance Use Disorders for Racial and Ethnic Minorities
Edited by Erick Guerrero and Tenie Khachikian
p. cm.
Print ISBN 978-1-78985-689-7
Online ISBN 978-1-78985-690-3
eBook (PDF) ISBN 978-1-78984-520-4

For EU product safety concerns:
IN TECH d.o.o., Prolaz Marije Krucifikse Kozulić 3, 51000 Rijeka, Croatia, info@intechopen.com or visit our website at intechopen.com.

Meet the editors

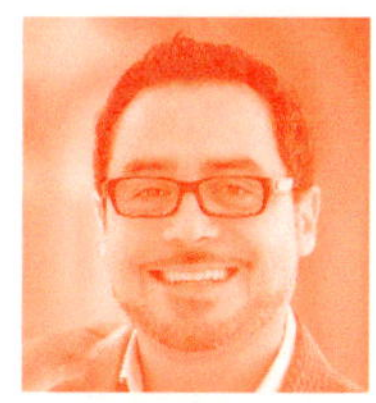

Erick Guerrero completed his doctoral degree at the University of Chicago in 2009. In 2016. Dr Guerrero received tenure as Associate Professor at the University of Southern California. Since 2018, he has been serving as the Founder and Director at the I-LEAD Institute, a research, consulting, and training firm. Dr Guerrero has a background in clinical psychology and organizational behavior. As a clinician, he has provided counseling to individuals, couples, and families for the past 23 years. As an organizational researcher, Dr Guerrero has published more than 60 peer-reviewed manuscripts and 2 books on implementation of evidence-based practices in human service organizations. Dr Guerrero currently leads international consortiums across several industries to help improve health care systems worldwide.

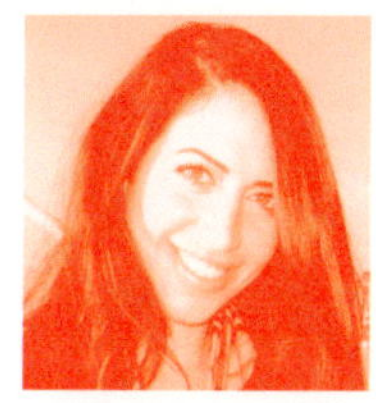

Tenie Khachikian received her PhD in Psychology at the University of California, Merced, in 2018. She has an M.S.W. in Social Work from the University of Southern California and her B.A. in Sociology from the University of California, Los Angeles. She has a background and experience in examining sociocultural factors particularly focused on health disparities and culturally responsive interventions. She has worked on several federally funded research studies that focus on improving health outcomes for racial and ethnic minority populations. During her doctoral program, she focused on exploring parent motivations to discuss unhealthy eating and marijuana use with their children, by developing and implementing health communications to motivate parent and child discussions on health-risk behaviors, in an effort to lessen these behaviors.

Contents

Preface

This book presents modifiable system level factors that may contribute to improving prevention and treatment of substance use disorders (SUD). The authors offer key insights on evidence-based interventions at the program and service delivery levels, particularly tailored to underserved population groups. For instance, the authors provide theory-based approaches to prevention (e.g. Familia Adelante), as well as spiritual, technical, and managerial approaches to treat SUDs and build capacity to deliver effective care. Overall, effective care in this book generally relates to delivering tested evidence-based practices (EBP) at the policy, management, and clinical service levels. The effective processes and practices that directly support the delivery of EBPs include case examples that invite reflection.

The idea for this book emerged from the growing need to understand how policy and management practices can support the effectiveness of clinical interventions. Most funding from government and private foundations is directed to randomized clinical trials in drug treatment, most of which are never implemented in regular care. Growing evidence suggests that building organizational capacity is necessary to improve fidelity in the implementation of EBPs resulting in greater effectiveness. The editors had two goals in mind for this book. First, to introduce to a wide audience promising modifiable factors that may improve systems of care, and second to invite policy and organizational scholars to expand on the proposed models and further examine how system factors can reduce the significant burden of substance abuse in our society.

We appreciate the thoughtful reviewers who made sure the contents of this book advance the state of knowledge. We are also thankful to colleagues who provided critical feedback throughout the chapter writing process. As editors, we are thankful to the authors included in this book for their significant contribution, and to their research assistants for supporting this effort.

Dr Guerrero is eternally grateful to his wife, Emma, and his two-year old daughter, Sophie, for their unconditional love and support, and for their encouragement to bring this book together. He is also thankful to the iSATed team for standing by him all these years and helping him and Dr Khachikian with this and other scholarly projects.

Dr Khachikian is first and foremost thankful to Dr Guerrero for inviting her to edit and contribute to this book alongside him. She would also like to thank her wonderful husband, Arnold, and her new bundle of joy, Aviana, for their support in completing this book.

Erick G. Guerrero, Ph.D.
I-Lead Institute,
Research to End Healthcare Disparities Corp,
Santa Monica, CA, USA

Tenie Khachikian, Ph.D., MSW
University of Chicago,
Chicago, IL, USA

Section 1

Introduction

Chapter 1

Introductory Chapter: Evidence-Based Practices to Improve Prevention and Treatment of Substance Use Disorders

Erick G. Guerrero and Tenie Khachikian

1. Introduction

Despite the significant burden of substance use disorders (SUD) across the world, SUD treatment systems face significant challenges to ensure immediate access to effective care. These systems are generally ill-equipped to respond to the unmet treatment needs of a population that is increasingly diverse in age, cultural, and linguistic background and in health severity. In the United States, 21 million people aged 12 or older needed SUD treatment in 2016, that is, 1 in 7 young adults and 6.9% of adults 26 or older [1]. The socioeconomic burden of SUD related to crime, lost work productivity, and healthcare amounts to 740 billion dollars a year [2], while the United States spends about 1.34 billion dollars a year in SUD prevention and 12.54 billion in SUD treatment a year [3]. Yet, only 1 out of 10 individuals seeking SUD treatment is able to access such care, and among those in treatments, fewer than 30% successfully complete their treatment episode. These alarming figures call for a comprehensive approach to improve the effectiveness of SUD treatment.

Prevention and treatment of SUDs in the United States is generally underfunded, and its effectiveness to reduce substance use is frequently questioned [4]. Although there are several evidence-based practices (EBPs) to prevent and treat SUDs, these practices are slowly disseminated through the system. One of the chief concerns to disseminate EBPs is the lack of system capacity to implement EBPs and with these efforts improve the effectiveness of care. Access to EBPs is the most challenging among low-income and racial/ethnic minority communities, which represent almost half of the individuals needing prevention and/or treatment [5].

2. Prevention

Despite the significant progress of prevention science in the past 20 years, there is limited knowledge of SUD prevention practices that work for non-White populations. This book focuses on one of the largest populations needing SUD prevention, Hispanic/Latinos. A growing literature is focusing on identifying and addressing risk and protective factors, such as acculturation stress, among others, that contributes to SUD among Latino adolescents. By understanding stress in relation to Latino's life in the United States, the proposed model in this book explains how discrimination, immigration, parent–child cultural differences, and other dynamics may trigger risk-taking behavior. The authors of the chapter on prevention propose a culturally focused prevention model, *Familia Adelante*, with significant empirical support to reduce substance use among Latinos.

3. Treatment

In the treatment section, we present innovative models to improve the effectiveness of SUD treatment. Although generally undermined, the use of spirituality and mindfulness in treatment has gained much attention. In this book, authors present a treatment model based on spirituality and culture to serve the needs of a growing culturally diverse population. Authors offer a nuanced discussion of the role of spirituality and mindfulness in contemporary treatment of addiction. Building from an integrated eclectic approach, authors propose a biopsychosocial-spiritual perspective. This chapter is written for both scientists and clinicians. By following the proposed model, authors provide both evidence-based and anecdotal experiences to draw in readers across several disciplines and perspectives. This approach is also included in the book because of its potential to engage clients in their recovery process and thus improve the effectiveness of treatment.

In this book, we also discuss leadership and management practices that indirectly support the effectiveness of SUD treatment systems. We generally focus on networks of treatment programs representing a large system of care. We lay a theoretical foundation of ways in which leadership and management may influence treatment staff (supervisors and counselors) to implement practices that enhance the effectiveness of care. The proposed conceptual model highlights how leadership, conceptualized as influence on employees to deliver quality of care, can be carried through managers at different levels. Because individuals within SUD treatment programs have different roles, responsibilities, and skills, it is important to understand how each of these individuals may be best motivated and prepared to implement culturally responsive and evidence-based care that enhances treatment effectiveness.

Preparing a workforce to effectively respond to the service needs of an increasingly diverse client population with co-occurring medical conditions requires significant investment in building knowledge, experience, and capacities. We place special attention to leadership development to prepare managers and treatment staff to understand organizational needs and functions and learn how to identify and modify factors that improve effectiveness. For instance, program leaders can learn how to build organizational development plans to diversify the workforce and ensure continuing technical support. Leaders can also establish succession planning and alignment to develop an organizational climate of trust and get buy-in from staff to implement specific EBPs. Investing in culturally responsive treatment is likely to improve treatment effectiveness.

We draw from the management literature to select critical evidence-based management practices (EBMPs) that may be feasible to implement in the SUD treatment system. We discuss EBMPs with different levels of complexity that require diverse levels of investment, in terms of technical assistance and other resources. These EBMPs can support the implementation of clinical EBPs and with those efforts improve the effectiveness of care. Many of these EBMPs could be adapted to effectively treat underserved populations, as described in the chapter on opioid treatment for African Americans.

Overall, the authors propose modifiable system and organizational-level factors that may improve the effectiveness of care, particularly for underserved populations. There is an immediate need for organizations to design and tailor their workforce to respond to the needs of culturally diverse populations in various arenas of healthcare. It is critical for policy makers, health administrators, program managers, and counselors to build on evidence-based management and leadership practices for successful prevention and treatment interventions that work. By delivering these practices, we could respond to the unmet treatment needs of the population we are serving and reduce the burden of SUD in our society.

Author details

Erick G. Guerrero[1]* and Tenie Khachikian[2]

1 I-Lead Institute, Research to End Healthcare Disparities Corp, Santa Monica, CA, USA

2 University of Chicago, Chicago, IL, USA

*Address all correspondence to: erickguerrero454@gmail.com

References

[1] Substance Abuse and Mental Health Services Administration. Key Substance Use and Mental Health Indicators in the United States: Results from the 2016 National Survey on Drug Use and Health (HHS Publication No. SMA 17-5044, NSDUH Series H-52). Rockville, MD: Center for Behavioral Health Statistics and Quality, Substance Abuse and Mental Health Services Administration; 2017. Available from: https://www.samhsa.gov/data/

[2] National Drug Intelligence Center. National Drug Threat Assessment. Washington, DC: United States Department of Justice; 2011. Available from: https://www.justice.gov/archive/ndic/pubs44/44848/44849p.pdf

[3] National Drug Control Budget: FY 2018 Funding Highlights. Washington, DC: Executive Office of the President, Office of National Drug Control Policy; 2017. Table 1, p. 16; Table 2, p. 18; and Table 3, p. 19. Available from: https://www.whitehouse.gov/sites/whitehouse.gov/files/ondcp/Fact_Sheets/FY2018-Budget-Highlights.pdf

[4] National Drug Control Budget: FY 2017 Funding Highlights. Washington, DC: Executive Office of the President, Office of National Drug Control Policy; 2016. Table 3, p. 19. Available from: https://www.whitehouse.gov/sites/whitehouse.gov/files/ondcp/Fact_Sheets/FY2018-Budget-Highlights.pdf

[5] Guerrero EG, Khachikian T, Frimpong JA, Kong Y, Howard DL, Hunter S. Drivers of continued implementation of cultural competence in substance use disorder treatment. Journal of Substance Abuse Treatment. 2019;**105**:5-11. DOI: 10.1016/j.jsat.2019.07.009

Section 2

Prevention

Chapter 2

Advances in Substance Abuse Prevention Practice and Science for Hispanic/Latinos

Richard C. Cervantes and Elias Koutantos

Abstract

The problem of substance abuse impacts the Hispanic/Latino youth population. In some cases, subpopulations of the Hispanic/Latino population suffer higher rates of substance use than do other groups. While the science of prevention in the general population and the rigorous study of substances abuse prevention programs have flourished over the past few decades, there continues to be a limited body of knowledge regarding substance abuse prevention that is culturally specific or tailored to Hispanic/Latinos. One promising area is the study of risk and protective factors which finds that acculturation stress, among others, plays a key role in the development of substance use and other behavioral problems among youth. Stress experiences related to discrimination, immigration, parent–child cultural differences all play a role in disrupting normative development and subsequent risk-taking behavior. Culturally focused prevention models such as *Familia Adelante* show promise in helping reduce acculturation-based risk and increasing individual and family resilience. This chapter will address many of the aforementioned issues and will provide direction for future prevention research for Hispanic/Latinos.

Keywords: Hispanic, substance abuse, prevention, acculturation, stress

1. Introduction

This chapter will provide an overview of substance use prevention for Hispanic/ Latino youth. Based on US Census Bureau data Hispanics are the youngest major racial or ethnic group in the United States [1]. About one-third or 17.9 million of the nation's Hispanic population is younger than 18 and about a quarter or 14.6 million of all Hispanics are millennials (ages 18–33 in 2014). Researchers and practitioners alike recognize the advantages of implementing prevention programming that averts the need for more intensive and costly drug treatments. Advances in prevention science have been highlighted in reports from the Institute of Medicine and National Institute on Drug Abuse (NIDA) among others. The question is whether such advances in scientifically based prevention efforts can also extend to Hispanic/ Latino youth including those who are immigrants or non-English speaking. A second question is whether theoretical models used to develop and study drug prevention programs are adequate in terms of addressing core cultural values beliefs and traditions among Hispanic/Latinos. Have prominent and widely used prevention interventions been adapted studied and proven effective with Hispanic/Latino youth? Are culturally tailored evidence-based programs available?

According to the review of literature conducted by Cuijpers [2], prevention programs have different goals, including the following: (a) increasing knowledge about drugs, (b) reducing the use, (c) delaying the onset of first use, (d) reducing abuse, and (e) minimizing the harm caused by the use. Prevention can be understood as any activity designed to avoid substance abuse and reduce its health and social consequences. This broad term can include actions aimed to reduce supply (e.g., based on the principle that the decreased availability of substances reduces the opportunities for abuse and dependence) and actions aimed to reduce demand (i.e., health promotion and disease prevention). In addition, the National Institute on Drug Abuse (NIDA), based on a growing body of prevention science, offers principles concerning prevention which range from the importance of addressing risk and protective factors to implementing and enforcing family and community policies prohibiting substance use [3]. Unfortunately, the NIDA principles do not specifically address the importance of cultural risk or protective factors that may impact substance use among Hispanics. Principle 12 does offer some broad recommendation regarding culture, citing that when communities adapt programs to match their needs, they should still do their best to maintain as close to the original intervention as possible and maintain high fidelity, although this principle is related to program adaptation.

2. Scope of the problem for Hispanic/Latino youth

Hispanic adolescents experience health disparities related to substance use, emotional problems, and high-risk sexual behavior. By the 12th grade, Latino students report the highest rates of 30-day use of marijuana, inhalants, ecstasy, cocaine, crack, salvia, Vicodin, methamphetamine, crystal methamphetamine, over-the-counter cough medicines, and tobacco through use of hookah [4]. Additionally, over one-quarter of Latino adolescents report alcohol use in the last 30 days as well as reports of the highest rates of binge and heavy drinking [5]. Suicide ideation is elevated among Latino adolescents as 1 in 7 (16.7%) Latino adolescents report suicidal ideation and 1in 10 (10.2%) report having attempted suicide [6]. In 2012, Latina adolescents had higher rates of teenage pregnancy than any other racial and ethnic minority, with 43.6 births per 1000 females, ages 15–19 years old [7].

The fastest-growing drug problem in the United States is prescription drugs, and it is profoundly affecting the lives of teenagers. According to NIDA DrugFacts, prescription drug misuse and abuse is when someone takes a medication inappropriately (e.g., without a prescription). According to National Survey on Drug Use and Health (NSDUH) data on youth and young adults, more than 5700 youth in 2014 reported using prescription pain relievers without a doctor's guidance for the first time.

A common misperception is that prescription drugs are safer or less harmful to one's body than other kinds of drugs. However, there are a range of short- and long-term health consequences for each type of prescription drugs used inappropriately. When concerning opioids, which act on the same parts of the brain as heroin, the consequences of inappropriate use can cause drowsiness, nausea, constipation, and depending on the amount taken, slowed breathing and even respiratory failure [8]. In terms of trends in tobacco use and electronic cigarettes among youth, older students, Hispanics, and Whites are more likely to use e-cigarettes than younger students and Blacks. In the young adult population, males, Hispanics, Whites, and those with lower education are more likely to use e-cigarettes than females, Blacks, and those with higher levels of education [9]. Flavored products marketed as e-cigarettes have gained popularity among youth and adults, while health consequence data continues to highlight the negative health impact of these products.

3. Risk and protective factors

Factors that drive the substance use behaviors of Hispanic youth may be quite similar to those found in the general population of youth, yet there are unique challenges, stressors, and other risk factors that play a role in the development of substance use among Hispanic/Latino youth [10]. Cultural values and language shifts, pre- and post-migration trauma, ethnic identified problems, and parent–child "acculturation gaps" are implicated in the onset of substance use in this growing population. A body of research on family stress, adaptation, and resilience by McCubbin and colleagues has established that stressors that impact minority groups, including Hispanics, can negatively impact and disrupt the family system [11]. In turn, how the family actively deals with their stressful conditions can strengthen family members, their relationships, and the family unit. Highly stressful conditions can overwhelm family functioning.

Acculturative stressors are a class of adverse conditions that can generate interpersonal, cultural and familial challenges. For example, cultural conflict following immigration can reverberate across generations. Such stressors may comprise chronic adversity that includes clashes between personal and family goals; an increase in individualistic views; a reduced sense of the importance of religion; increased intra-family conflicts; gender role conflict; and increased marital conflict. Families with more acculturative stress and who lack a strong social support system or resilience (i.e., family and friends, spiritual resources, access to public social services) or personal resources (i.e., self-esteem) can show a greater decline in family cohesion.

4. Immigration and acculturation-related hardships confronted by Hispanic/Latino youth

The physical and emotional demands of immigrating to the United States are well documented [12]. New data shows a 117% increase in unaccompanied children ages 12 and under caught at the US-Mexico border in fiscal year 2014 compared to fiscal year 2013. By comparison, the number of apprehensions of children 13–17 years old has by increased 12% in the past year [13]. Parental deportation is an increasingly common hardship experienced by the Hispanic youth. Nearly 33,000 noncitizen youth are in DHS custody each day, representing an over 50% increase from 2001. Chaudry and colleagues found most children of deported undocumented workers remained in the United States with their other parent or relative [14]. The negative consequences of forced family separation because of deportation on child well-being are documented [15–18]. Children most at risk for negative behavioral or psychological changes are those who witnessed their parents' arrest; children separated from their parents longer than 30 days; and children whose primary caregiver was deported [19].

The term *acculturative stress* refers to the distress that individuals experience as a result of tension between maintaining the behaviors and characteristics of their country of origin and concurrently adopting those from the majority culture [20]. Acculturative stressors are not unique to Latino populations and may include pressure from learning a new language, balancing differences in cultural values, and adjusting to new employment expectations [21, 22]. Stress itself is conceptualized as a behavioral and emotional reaction to acute or chronic life-changing events and occurs when the demands of the events exceed the individuals' perceived personal and social resources to deal with these changes [23]. The stress-illness paradigm offers one way to conceptualize the relationship between social stress and health [24, 25].

Research studies on acculturation and health status have been mixed, with some studies showing a positive relation between acculturation and health, while others demonstrate an inverse effect on health outcomes [26]. Furthermore, there is often considerable variation in these outcomes depending on factors such as country of origin, age, gender, years lived in the United States, education, and income [27]. For example, some research shows differences in health outcomes across a number of Latino/a subpopulations, with some subgroups experiencing higher morbidity and mortality rates, diabetes and hypertension, psychiatric disorders, and substance use disorders [27–32]. One potential factor driving these different outcomes is experiences of acculturative stress.

Recent work by the authors suggests that acculturation "gaps" between adolescents and their parents can impact healthy emotional development. An additional adversity often faced by Hispanic families involves family member separations due to immigration, such as when parents come to the United States first and children are separated for years. The reunification process can be stressful and painful rather than smooth and joyous. The work by Perreira and colleagues emphasizes how adversity and resilient responses are embedded in social contexts. From an adversities' perspective, this involves loss of social position and class status, loss of vital extended family resources, loss of peer networks and community support, and economic and social segregation and marginalization. Unfamiliar social contexts, language barriers, and humiliation when confronted by racism and discrimination can further erode individual and family coping and resilience.

Studies also indicate that US-born and more acculturated Mexican origin youth exhibit higher rates of externalizing behavior when compared to their less acculturated, Mexican-born peers. Markers of acculturation are consistently associated with externalizing outcomes like conduct problems, juvenile arrest, and substance use. US-born youth report less investment in education and lower academic aspirations than their Mexican-born peers [33]. Among immigrants, greater length of residence in the United States is associated with lowered academic motivation [34, 35]. Despite the stressful period of adjustment to a new set of cultural and linguistic changes, immigrants show resilience and better behavioral health compared to US-born Latino youth. The immigrant paradox primarily results from the progressive loss of traditional culture and associated negative health consequences associated with increasing generations or time in the United States [36].

Research examining the effects of both acculturation and stress find that stress partially mediates the relationship between acculturation and negative health behaviors. Stress impedes health by limiting access to salutogenic health behaviors and through maladaptive coping [37]. Hispanics under elevated stressor exposure are more likely to deny the stressor or to use maladaptive coping behaviors such as risky sex and substance abuse [38, 39].

Among youth, immigration, and acculturation-related stressors have also been found to predict greater drug use and risky sexual behavior [40, 41]. Recently, Cervantes and colleagues identified eight culturally based stress risk domains commonly experienced by Latino adolescents, ranging from acculturation gaps to family immigration-related stress [42]. Higher scores of cultural stress in these life domains were significantly related to both internalizing and externalizing behavioral health problems in Latino adolescents including polysubstance use [10, 42]. Effective interventions targeting immigration-related stress among Hispanics must promote healthy coping strategies for acculturation- and immigration-based stressors [43].

The implications of immigration and acculturation stressors are likely accentuated in new Hispanic settlement communities. New settlement areas are often hostile towards immigrants, creating a culture of fear where there is a heightened sense of anxiety that likely underlies social interaction and exaggerates possible stressor exposure. Birman and colleagues provide evidence that these hostile contextual conditions can affect the acculturation process and point to contextual factors such as immigrant density, acceptance of cultural diversity, and presence of social capital as core contextual issues [44].

5. Protective effects of family and social support

Protective factors are those personal and environmental conditions and experiences that can counteract risk factors for substance use. For example, emphasis on family life is a central core value to most Hispanics and essential for their resilience in achieving normative life aims in the face of adverse social and environmental barriers. The concept of *familismo*/familism is a core value and belief in the centrality of family in the life of Hispanics. It highlights family loyalty, interdependence over independence, and cooperation over competition. Hispanic cultural values (i.e., *familismo*, *simpatia*, power distance, personal space, present time orientation, traditional gender roles) may impact health outcomes and diminish during the acculturation process. Embracing familism as a value contributes to a familial stability, which is linked to better physical health behaviors,

Acculturation risk factors	Suggested resilience strategies
Discrimination	• Maintaining a strong sense of identity and self-confidence • Demonstrating strong sense of cultural identity • Leaning towards religion and spirituality to assist emotions when dealing with discrimination • Finding resources voting for beneficial measures and laws
Immigration stress	• Becoming educated on the topic of immigration • Take ESL classes • Maintaining hope towards the future and focusing on the positive aspects of immigration • Finding assistance through ESL and studying • Relying on the bible to maintain hope
Family conflicts	• Seeking support from other family members • Spirituality and seeking help from God and clergy • Increasing communication skills with family
Health-related stress	• Seeking traditional remedies • Getting help from pharmacies that have meds from other countries (e.g., going to Mexico) • Finding local clinics and low-income assistance clinics • Relying on family for emotional and monetary support • Dev eloping healthier habits to prevent health problems
Marital problems	• Learning from others.; asking for advice • Seeking assistance from other family members or clergy

Table 1.
Protective factors and resilience strategies.

higher likelihood of seeking medical help, better psychological health, and lower perceived burden of stress.

Familism and the highly involved parenting practices that often come with familism have been linked to fewer behavior problems in children. The work by Perreira and colleagues has pointed to specific resiliency strategies utilized by Hispanic immigrant parents. These include (1) emphasizing with and respecting adolescents/children (i.e., developing a deep understanding of what they are going through in an unfamiliar context and admiring the strength shown by children in that difficult context); (2) seeking help and fostering social support (i.e., connecting to other Hispanics and building community); (3) developing bicultural coping skills (including teaching children about their heritage and American culture); and (4) improving communication with their children (e.g., speaking honestly about difficult situations and being attentive to the child's needs). *Familismo*, the orientation towards putting the needs of the family above that of the individual, family cohesiveness, reciprocity, and honor is a core value in Hispanic/Latino culture [45–49]. Most studies of psychosocial outcomes related to *familismo* find favorable psychosocial results for Hispanic children and adolescents [50–55]. Incorporating Hispanic/Latino family values into early intervention and prevention programs can buffer the impact of weakening connection to traditional family protective factors [56].

Other forms of resilience can be found among Hispanic/Latino youth and families. These resources can be "mobilized" as part of any culturally focused prevention strategy. In one qualitative study of family resilience, Cervantes and Santisteban [57] reported specific, contextual resilience strategies mentioned by Hispanic/Latino families in confronting acculturation stressors (**Table 1**).

6. Research on behavioral intervention strategies for Hispanic/Latino youth

Evidence-based drug prevention programming for Hispanic/Latinos does exist, although the number or programs is small. Familias Unidas, Familia Adelante, Strengthening the Bonds of Chicano Youth, and other similar programs will be highlighted here. The *Familias Unidas* intervention research has been undertaken with various Hispanic/Latino population groups including a study of predominantly Cuban (39%), Central and South Americans (29 and 17%, respectively), and a small proportion of Puerto Rican/Dominican (5%) participants [58]. A more recent study of *Familias Unidas* included adolescent participants who were predominantly US-born (56.1%) as well as adolescent immigrants from Honduras (26.9%), Cuba (20.4%), and Nicaragua (16.1%) [59]. A study of *Strengthening the Bonds of Chicano Youth* (El Proyecto de Nuestra Juventud) included 450 high-risk youth in an established, nonimmigrant community setting [60]. Results were generally positive in reducing risk factors for substance use.

Familias Preparando la Nueva Generación (FPNG) is a synchronized culturally grounded parenting component program which involves Latino youth substance abuse prevention [61]. FPNG serves as an addition to the already proven efficacious classroom-based drug abuse prevention intervention, Keepin' it Real (KIR). One study showed that anti-drug norms were stronger in participants who were enrolled in KIR whose parents also participated in FPNG than in participants who were enrolled in KIR alone. Along with these stronger anti-drug norms, participants whose parents were in FPNG also showed reduced use of cigarettes and alcohol. The findings have shown that adolescent normative beliefs and related behaviors can be changed through synchronized culturally grounded parent and youth interventions.

REAL Groups is a small-group intervention designed to complement the school-based Keepin' it Real (KIR) prevention program [62]. REAL Groups intervention is the result of a partnership with predominantly Mexican-American schools located in the central city neighborhoods of a southwestern US metropolitan area. The REAL Groups approach was designed as a companion to the larger KIR intervention and takes place over 10 weeks specifically targeting Latino, Hispanic, and Mexican-American children that appear to be more vulnerable to using drugs before entering adolescence. However, the outcomes of the REAL Groups intervention have been mixed and inconclusive, mainly due to the participants of the study being in the fifth grade with low drug use rates.

The mother/daughter intervention (MDI) approach is another program that involves substance abuse prevention strategies for youth [63]. This approach consists of 10 sessions via the internet which are to be completed at a rate of one session per week. In one study the MDI targeted young Black and Latina girls between the ages of 10 and 13 and their mothers. The outcome of the MDI showed that the girls who received the intervention reported lower levels of depression and higher levels of self-efficacy about their ability to avoid cigarette smoking, alcohol consumption, and drug use.

Substance abuse treatment and prevention interventions also exist to address intrafamilial stress in Hispanic families, such as brief strategic family therapy (BSFT) and more recently culturally informed family therapy for adolescents (CIFTA) [64, 65]. Again, these studies have included predominately Cuban or other Caribbean Latino samples yet may prove beneficial when applied to other Hispanic/Latino groups.

7. Integrating acculturation stress into prevention efforts

As an example of the expanding set of innovative research-based prevention programs for Hispanic/Latino youth, Familia Adelante will be will be discussed in some detail to exemplify one recently developed, culturally focused program. Familia Adelante is a drug prevention program that incorporates *promotores* as facilitators for this curriculum-based drug prevention program. The first iteration of the *Familia Adelante* (FA) curriculum showed reductions in family stress

	Familia adelante: youth sessions summary	
Session	**Lesson**	**Lesson goal**
1	Introduction	Have a clear understanding of the Familia adelante curriculum, its purpose, and the need for program evaluation
2	Concept building	To define prevention and its application in life, build rapport with group members, acknowledge Hispanic culture as a positive resiliency factor, learn the basic concepts of culture and stress
3	Feelings	Explore physical and emotional feelings, explain how feelings affect behavior; how to be assertive in relationships
4	Stress overview	What stress is and how it affects physical and emotional health as well as behavior
5	Acculturation stress	Hispanic acculturation stress, how to identify the consequences of physical and emotional stress, and what values may hold. Discussion of immigration-related stressors
6	School-related stress	Identify the stressors related to school, cultural, and ethnic differences and how this stress affects youth; help youth identify trusted adults to share stressful experiences

	Familia adelante: youth sessions summary	
Session	**Lesson**	**Lesson goal**
7	Negative peer pressure	Adaptive ways of coping with stress; how to cope with dating peer pressure around sexual behaviors.
8	Family stress	How to identify family stressors; effective ways to deal with cultural stressors, positive and negatives about having sex; explore acculturation gaps
9	Gang prevention	Understand Hispanic gangs, violence, and the importance of not becoming members of gangs
10	Substance abuse education	Specific drug information, dangers of drug use, other healthy activities, facts about drugs, effects of drugs on a person's body, cultural pressures to use alcohol and other drugs
11	Family communication	Teach families healthy communication skills; revisit acculturation gaps stressors
12	Evaluation and celebration	Re-evaluate youth to assess effectiveness of program; certificates of completion awarded to participants

Table 2.
Familia adelante session summary.

and youth behavior problems, enhancing academic and psychosocial coping and decreasing substance use patterns in Latino youth [66]. FA was also tested through in the SAMHSA-funded Blythe Street Prevention Project (BSPP) with youth and their parents, and that study found significant improvements in drug knowledge and drug resistance skills in both youth and parents [67]. *FA* was then evaluated in 2006 with six cohorts of families in a school-based setting. Findings were positive showing that family and peer communication improved and perceptions of substance use harm increased while social norms around sexual behavior and past-30-day use of marijuana and illegal drugs were reduced [68]. The developers also conducted NIH-supported work to infuse the *FA* curriculum with reproductive health education and HIV prevention messaging. Based on focus group data, new content was identified by participating youth that was not included in the original *FA* curriculum (i.e., content on eating disorders) (**Table 2**).

8. Adapting evidence-based programs

Given the lack of prevention programs that have used a grounded cultural theory or that have incorporated culturally relevant risk and protective factors, there is oftentimes a need to use other evidence-based prevention practices and approaches and to adapt those to the needs of local Hispanic/Latino community. In one literature review comparing cultural adaptations to either no treatment or unadapted treatments, researchers found that cultural adaptations can be more effective than either of these other conditions, especially for clients with a diagnosed mental health disorder [69]. When examined as a whole, the scientific literature on cultural adaptations shows treatment effects to be significant and moderate in size on average [69–75]. Still, researchers caution that conclusions about the need for cultural adaptations should be reserved until more studies that directly compare adapted and unadapted EBPPs are conducted.

Adapted interventions that address the powerful, everyday stressors experienced by Hispanic/Latino clients are likely to be perceived as more relevant and attractive to clients. Enhancing content of existing EBPPs to reflect the values (e.g., family, religion) and world views of Latino clients will also increase the cultural relevance of the intervention [69, 76]. Finally, there are a number of agency- and provider-level characteristics that must be considered before a decision to adapt an EBP is made. First and foremost is the capacity of a provider organization to systematically undertake an adaptation. Agency capacity refers to the financial and human capital resources, skills, knowledge, and in-kind support that are needed to take on each step of the adaptation process (outlined below). For example, an initial needs assessment may include conducting consumer, staff, and other stakeholder interviews or focus groups. Thus, an agency should be prepared to cover costs related to staffing of these additional activities, paying incentives for participants, offering childcare, providing food and providing transportation for participants, transcription of focus group data, data management, data analysis, and reporting.

9. Conclusions and recommendations for future research

Drug prevention science and practice continues to expand, and to some extent the field has made positive impact in the Hispanic/Latino community. Based on the research to date, sufficient evidence exists about culturally specific risk and protective factors associated with the onset of substance use [3, 42]. Additionally, the momentum is gathering for the development and study of culturally focused prevention interventions. Acculturation and related stressors have been shown to precipitate behavioral health problems, and the body of research on acculturation stress can serve as theoretical underpinnings for the development of additional contemporary, culturally sensitive programming. As prevention programming and the evidence base for Hispanic/Latino practices continues to expand, core theoretical considerations will drive effective prevention programming. Latino and other scholars agree that concepts of acculturation, acculturation stress, familismo, *respeto*, and *comunidad* (community) must be inherent components, if not core components of prevention strategies for this growing population. Reinforcing positive family and youth identity that incorporates, embraces, and honors cultural history and traditions appears to have most promise.

In addition, there is growing evidence that factors such as acculturation stress, parent–child acculturation gaps, and prolonged discrimination (measured by allostatic load) may all play a role in the development of SUD among Hispanic/Latino youth. Programs such as Familia Adelante, which can be considered a culturally grounded model, address many of the acculturation and stress-related issues that resonate with many Hispanic/Latino youth. The development of prevention service approaches that include family and parent involvement is necessary, not only for the purpose of recruiting and retaining families but also as a way to promote and reinforce *familismo*. Future research on the impact of immigration policy and enforcement is needed particularly related to how family separations, childhood trauma associated with immigration, and deportation experiences lead to the development of behavioral health problems. The testing of prevention programs that are specific to new immigrants and refugee populations will be needed to address the uncertainties that these youth and families experience and that may not be addressed in existing prevention models.

Finally, we have outlined issues related to adapting existing EPBs for use in Hispanic/Latino communities. Research is fairly conclusive that adapting an EBP to the language and cultural characteristics of a particular ethnic community is better than not doing the adaption. Yet, the skills, capacity, and resources available to do good program adaptation must be in place. More specific research on program adaptations of generic prevention programs for Hispanic/Latino communities is needed.

Author details

Richard C. Cervantes* and Elias Koutantos
Behavioral Assessment Inc., Los Angeles, California, USA

*Address all correspondence to: rccbeth@aol.com

References

[1] US Census Bureau. The Hispanic Population in the United States: 2014. The United States Census Bureau. Available from: https://www.census.gov/data/tables/2014/demo/hispanic-origin/2014-cps.html. Published August 23 2017. Accessed [December 10 2019]

[2] Cuijpers P. Three decades of drug prevention research. Drugs: Education, Prevention and Policy. 2003;**10**(1):7-20. DOI: 10.1080/0968763021000018900

[3] Releases IOM. Report on preventing mental, emotional, and behavioral disorders among young people: progress and possibilities. Journal of Child and Adolescent Psychiatric Nursing. 2010;**23**(2):118-118. DOI: 10.1111/j.1744-6171.2010.00231.x

[4] Johnston L, Miech R, Omalley P, Bachman J, Schulenberg J, Patrick M. Monitoring the Future national survey results on drug use, 1975-2017: Overview, key findings on adolescent drug use. Ann Arbor: Institute for Social Research, University of Michigan; 2018. DOI: 10.3998/2027.42/148123

[5] Pemberton MR, Colliver JD, Robbins TM, Gfroerer JC. Underage alcohol use: Findings from the 2002-2006 national surveys on drug use and health. PsycEXTRA Dataset. Rockville, MD: Substance Abuse and Mental Health Services Administration, Office of Applied Studies; 2008. DOI: 10.1037/e474852008-001. DHHS Publication No. SMA 08-4333, Analytic Series A-30

[6] Youth Risk Behavior Surveillance. United States: Centers for Disease Control and Prevention; 2011. Available from: https://www.cdc.gov/mmwr/preview/mmwrhtml/ss6104a1.htm?s_cid=ss6104a1_w. Accessed [December 12 2019]

[7] Martin JA, Hamilton BE, Ventura SJ, Osterman MJK, Matthews TJ. Births: Final Data for 2011. Centers for Disease Control and Prevention. Available from: https://stacks.cdc.gov/view/cdc/23435. Published June 28 2013. Accessed [December 12 2019]

[8] Volk K. Teen Prescription Drug Misuse and Abuse. SAMHSA. 2019. Available from: https://www.samhsa.gov/homelessness-programs-resources/hpr-resources/teen-prescription-drug-misuse-abuse [Accessed: October 21, 2019]

[9] U.S. Department of Health and Human Services. E-Cigarette Use Among Youth and Young Adults: A Report of the Surgeon General-Executive Summary. Atlanta, GA: U.S. Department of Health and Human Services, Centers for Disease Control and Prevention, National Center for Chronic Disease Prevention and Health Promotion, Office on Smoking and Health; 2016

[10] Cardoso JB, Goldbach JT, Cervantes RC, Swank P. Stress and multiple substance use behaviors among Hispanic adolescents. Prevention Science. 2015;**17**(2):208-217. DOI: 10.1007/s11121-015-0603-6

[11] McCubbin HI, Thompson AI, McCubbin MA. Family Assessment: Resiliency, Coping and Adaptation: Inventories for Research and Practice. Madison, WI: University of Wisconsin Publishers; 1997

[12] Patten E. The Nation's Latino Population Is Defined by Its Youth. Pew Research Center's Hispanic Trends Project. 2016. Available from: https://www.pewresearch.org/hispanic/2016/04/20/the-nations-latino-population-is-defined-by-its-youth/ [Accessed: October 11, 2019]

[13] Krogstad JM, Keegan M. 15 States with the Highest Share of

Immigrants in Their Population. Pew Research Center. 2014. Available from: https://www.pewresearch.org/fact-tank/2014/05/14/15-states-with-the-highest-share-of-immigrants-in-their-population/ [Accessed: October 21, 2019]

[14] Chaudry A, Capps R, Pedroza JM, Castaneda RM, Santos R, Scott MM. Facing our future: Children in the aftermath of immigration enforcement. Research Report. Urban Institute. 2010. DOI: 10.1037/e726272011-001

[15] Capps R. Paying the Price: The Impact of Immigration Raids on Americas Children. National Council of La Raza: Washington, D.C; 2007

[16] Fortuny K, Capps R, Simms M, Chaudry A. Children of immigrants: National and state characteristics. Research Report. Urban Institute. 2009. DOI: 10.1037/e724062011-001

[17] Hondagneu-Sotelo P, Avila E. Im here, but Im there. Gender and Society. 1997;**11**(5):548-571. DOI: 10.1177/089124397011005003

[18] Suarez-Orozco C, Todorova IL, Louie J. Making up for lost time: The experience of separation and reunification among immigrant families. Family Process. 2002;**41**(4):625-643. DOI: 10.1111/j.1545-5300.2002.00625.x

[19] Fortuny K, Chaudry A. A Comprehensive Review of Immigrant Access to Health and Human Services. 2011. Available from: https://www.urban.org/research/publication/comprehensive-review-immigrant-access-health-and-human-services/view/full_report

[20] Cervantes RC, Castro FG. Stress, coping, and Mexican American mental health: A systematic review. Hispanic Journal of Behavioral Sciences. 1985;7(1):1-73. DOI: 10.1177/07399863850071001

[21] Araújo BY, Borrell LN. Understanding the link between discrimination, mental health outcomes, and life chances among Latinos. Hispanic Journal of Behavioral Sciences. 2006;**28**(2):245-266. DOI: 10.1177/0739986305285825

[22] Torres L, Driscoll MW, Voell M. Discrimination, acculturation, acculturative stress, and Latino psychological distress: A moderated mediational model. Cultural Diversity & Ethnic Minority Psychology. 2012;**18**(1):17-25. DOI: 10.1037/a0026710

[23] Lazarus RS, Folkman S. Stress, Appraisal, and Coping. New York: Springer Pub. Co.; 1984

[24] Ensel WM. "important" life events and depression among older adults. Journal of Aging and Health. 1991;**3**(4):546-566. DOI: 10.1177/089826439100300407

[25] Pearlin LI. The sociological study of stress. Journal of Health and Social Behavior. 1989;**30**(3):241. DOI: 10.2307/2136956

[26] Hunt LM, Schneider S, Comer B. Should “acculturation” be a variable in health research? A critical review of research on US Hispanics. Social Science & Medicine. 2004;**59**(5):973-986. DOI: 10.1016/j.socscimed.2003.12.009

[27] Lara M, Gamboa C, Kahramanian MI, Morales LS, Bautista DEH. Acculturation and Latino health in the United States: A review of the literature and its sociopolitical context. Annual Review of Public Health. 2005;**26**(1):367-397.

DOI: 10.1146/annurev.publhealth.26.021304.144615

[28] Martinez-Tyson D, Pathak EB, Soler-Vila H, Flores AM. Looking under the Hispanic umbrella: Cancer mortality among Cubans, Mexicans, Puerto Ricans and other Hispanics in Florida. Journal of Immigrant and Minority Health. 2008;**11**(4):249-257. DOI: 10.1007/s10903-008-9152-4

[29] Arroyo-Johnson C, Mincey KD, Ackermann N, Milam L, Goodman MS, Colditz GA. Racial and ethnic heterogeneity in self-reported diabetes prevalence trends across Hispanic subgroups, national health interview survey, 1997-2012. Preventing Chronic Disease. 2016;**13**. Available from: http://dx.doi.org/ 10.5888/pcd13.150260. Published January 21 2016. [Accessed: December 12 2019]

[30] Pabon-Nau LP, Cohen A, Meigs JB, Grant RW. Hypertension and diabetes prevalence among U.S. Hispanics by country of origin: The national health interview survey 2000-2005. Journal of General Internal Medicine. 2010;**25**(8):847-852. DOI: 10.1007/s11606-010-1335-8

[31] Alegria M, Canino G, Stinson FS, Grant BF. Nativity and DSM-IV psychiatric disorders among Puerto Ricans, Cuban Americans, and non-Latino whites in the United States. The Journal of Clinical Psychiatry. 2006;**67**(1):56-65. DOI: 10.4088/jcp.v67n0109

[32] Alegría M, Canino G, Shrout PE, et al. Prevalence of mental illness in immigrant and non-immigrant U.S. Latino groups. The American Journal of Psychiatry. 2008;**165**(3):359-369. DOI: 10.1176/appi.ajp.2007.07040704

[33] Fuligni AJ, Eccles JS, Barber BL, Clements P. Early adolescent peer orientation and adjustment during high school. Developmental Psychology. 2001;**37**(1):28-36. DOI: 10.1037//0012-1649.37.1.28

[34] Carola S-O, Suárez-Orozco Marcelo M. Children of Immigration. Cambridge: Harvard University Press; 2001

[35] Portes A, Rumbaut Rubén G. Legacies: The Story of the Immigrant Second Generation. Berkeley, CA: University of California Press;

[36] Vega WA, Rodriguez MA, Gruskin E. Health disparities in the Latino population. Epidemiologic Reviews. 2009;**31**(1):99-112. DOI: 10.1093/epirev/mxp008

[37] Allen JD, Caspi C, Yang M, Leyva B, Stoddard AM, Tamers S, et al. Pathways between acculturation and health behaviors among residents of low-income housing: The mediating role of social and contextual factors. Social Science & Medicine. 2014;**123**:26-36. DOI: 10.1016/j.socscimed.2014.10.034

[38] Perez SM, Gavin JK, Diaz VA. Stressors and coping mechanisms associated with perceived stress in Latinos. Ethnicity & Disease. 2015;**25**(1):78-82

[39] Cummings AM, Gonzalez-Guarda RM, Sandoval MF. Intimate partner violence among Hispanics: A review of the literature. Journal of Family Violence. 2012;**28**(2):153-171. DOI: 10.1007/s10896-012-9478-5

[40] Martinez CR. Effects of differential family acculturation on Latino adolescent substance use. Family Relations. 2006;**55**(3):306-317. DOI: 10.1111/j.1741-3729.2006.00404.x

[41] Levy V, Page-Shafer K, Evans J, et al. HIV-related risk behavior among Hispanic immigrant men in a population-based household survey in

low-income neighborhoods of northern California. Sexually Transmitted Diseases. 2005;**32**(8):487-490. DOI: 10.1097/01.olq.0000161185.06387.94

[42] Cervantes RC, Fisher DG, Córdova D, Napper LE. The Hispanic stress inventory—Adolescent version: A culturally informed psychosocial assessment. Psychological Assessment. 2012;**24**(1):187-196. DOI: 10.1037/a0025280

[43] Cervantes RC, Fisher DG, Padilla AM, Napper LE. The Hispanic stress inventory version 2: Improving the assessment of acculturation stress. Psychological Assessment. 2016;**28**(5):509-522. DOI: 10.1037/pas0000200

[44] Birman D, Trickett E, Buchanan RM. A tale of two cities: Replication of a study on the acculturation and adaptation of immigrant adolescents from the former Soviet Union in a different community context. American Journal of Community Psychology. 2005;**35**(1-2):83-101. DOI: 10.1007/s10464-005-1891-y

[45] Steidel AGL, Contreras JM. A new familism scale for use with Latino populations. Hispanic Journal of Behavioral Sciences. 2003;**25**(3):312-330. DOI: 10.1177/0739986303256912

[46] Marin G, Sabogal F, Marin BV, Otero-Sabogal R, Perez-Stable EJ. Development of a short acculturation scale for Hispanics. Hispanic Journal of Behavioral Sciences. 1987;**9**(2):183-205. DOI: 10.1177/07399863870092005

[47] Zinn MB. Chicano men and masculinity. Journal of Ethnic Studies. 1982;**10**(2):29-44

[48] Comeau JA. Race/ethnicity and family contact. Hispanic Journal of Behavioral Sciences. 2012;**34**(2):251-268. DOI: 10.1177/0739986311435899

[49] Falicov CJ. Working with transnational immigrants: Expanding meanings of family, community, and culture. Family Process. 2007;**46**(2):157-171. DOI: 10.1111/j.1545-5300.2007.00201.x

[50] Calderón-Tena CO, Knight GP, Carlo G. The socialization of prosocial behavioral tendencies among Mexican American adolescents: The role of familism values. Cultural Diversity & Ethnic Minority Psychology. 2011;**17**(1):98-106. DOI: 10.1037/a0021825

[51] Morcillo C, Duarte CS, Shen S, Blanco C, Canino G, Bird HR. Parental familism and antisocial behaviors: Development, gender, and potential mechanisms. Journal of the American Academy of Child and Adolescent Psychiatry. 2011;**50**(5):471-479. DOI: 10.1016/j.jaac.2011.01.014

[52] Esparza P, Sánchez B. The role of attitudinal familism in academic outcomes: A study of urban, Latino high school seniors. Cultural Diversity & Ethnic Minority Psychology. 2008;**14**(3):193-200. DOI: 10.1037/1099-9809.14.3.193

[53] Germán M, Gonzales NA, Dumka L. Familism values as a protective factor for Mexican-origin adolescents exposed to deviant peers. The Journal of Early Adolescence. 2008;**29**(1):16-42. DOI: 10.1177/0272431608324475

[54] Kuperminc GP, Wilkins NJ, Jurkovic GJ, Perilla JL. Filial responsibility, perceived fairness, and psychological functioning of Latino youth from immigrant families. Journal of Family Psychology. 2013;**27**(2):173-182. DOI: 10.1037/a0031880

[55] Marsiglia FF, Parsai M, Kulis S. Effects of familism and family cohesion on problem behaviors among adolescents in Mexican immigrant families in the Southwest United States.

Journal of Ethnic and Cultural Diversity in Social Work. 2009;**18**(3):203-220. DOI: 10.1080/15313200903070965

[56] Castro FG, Barrera JM, Martinez JCR. The Cultural Adaptation of Prevention Interventions: Resolving Tensions Between Fidelity and Fit. Prevention Science. 2004;**5**(1):41-45. DOI:10.1023/b:prev.0000013980.12412.cd

[57] Cervantes RC, Santisteban DS. Enhancing family resilience among at risk Latinos panel presentation. In: Presented at the Society for Prevention Research Annual Conference, San Francisco, CA. 2016

[58] Pantin H, Schwartz SJ, Sullivan S, Coatsworth JD, Szapocznik J. Preventing substance abuse in Hispanic immigrant adolescents: An ecodevelopmental, parent-centered approach. Hispanic Journal of Behavioral Sciences. 2003;**25**(4):469-500. DOI: 10.1177/0739986303259355

[59] Pantin H, Prado G, Lopez B, et al. A randomized controlled trial of familias unidas for Hispanic adolescents with behavior problems. Psychosomatic Medicine. 2009;**71**(9):987-995. DOI: 10.1097/psy.0b013e3181bb2913

[60] Varela R. Cultural Competent Prevention Program for At-Risk Chicano Youth. Substance Abuse Mental Health Services Administration/Center for Substance Abuse Prevention (SAMHSA/CSAP) Report. Washington, DC: Samhsa, Csap, U.S. Department of Health and Human Services; 2001

[61] Marsiglia FF, Ayers SL, Baldwin-White A, Booth J. Changing Latino adolescents' substance use norms and behaviors: The effects of synchronized youth and parent drug use prevention interventions. Prevention Science. 2015;**17**(1):1-12. DOI: 10.1007/s11121-015-0574-7

[62] Marsiglia FF, Peña V, Nieri T, Nagoshi JL. Real groups: The design and immediate effects of a prevention intervention for Latino children. Social Work With Groups. 2010;**33**(2-3):103-121. DOI: 10.1080/01609510903366202

[63] Schinke SP, Fang L, Cole KC, Cohen-Cutler S. Preventing substance use among black and Hispanic adolescent girls: Results from a computer-delivered, mother–daughter intervention approach. Substance Use & Misuse. 2010;**46**(1):35-45. DOI: 10.3109/10826084.2011.521074

[64] Santisteban DA, Coatsworth JD, Perez-Vidal A, et al. Efficacy of brief strategic family therapy in modifying Hispanic adolescent behavior problems and substance use. Journal of Family Psychology. 2003;**17**(1):121-133. DOI: 10.1037//0893-3200.17.1.121

[65] Santisteban DA, Mena MP, Mccabe BE. Preliminary results for an adaptive family treatment for drug abuse in Hispanic youth. Journal of Family Psychology. 2011;**25**(4):610-614. DOI: 10.1037/a0024016

[66] Cervantes R, Goldbach J, Santos SM. Familia adelante: A multi-risk prevention intervention for Latino families. The Journal of Primary Prevention. 2011;**32**(3-4):225-234. DOI: 10.1007/s10935-011-0251-y

[67] Cervantes RC, Pena C. Evaluating Hispanic/Latino programs. Alcoholism Treatment Quarterly. 1998;**16**(1-2):109-131. DOI: 10.1300/j020v16n01_07

[68] Bernal G, Adames C. Cultural adaptations: Conceptual, ethical, contextual, and methodological issues for working with ethnocultural and majority-world populations. Prevention Science. 2017;**18**(6):681-688. DOI: 10.1007/s11121-017-0806-0

[69] Hall GCN, Ibaraki AY, Huang ER, Marti CN, Stice E. A meta-analysis of cultural adaptations of psychological interventions. Behavior Therapy.

2016;**47**(6):993-1014. DOI: 10.1016/j.beth.2016.09.005

[70] Benish SG, Quintana S, Wampold BE. Culturally adapted psychotherapy and the legitimacy of myth: A direct-comparison meta-analysis. Journal of Counseling Psychology. 2011;**58**(3):279-289. DOI: 10.1037/a0023626

[71] Griner D, Smith TB. Culturally adapted mental health intervention: A meta-analytic review. Psychotherapy: Theory, Research, Practice, Training. 2006;**43**(4):531-548. DOI: 10.1037/0033-3204.43.4.531

[72] Huey SJ, Polo AJ. Evidence-based psychosocial treatments for ethnic minority youth. Journal of Clinical Child and Adolescent Psychology. 2008;**37**(1):262-301. DOI: 10.1080/15374410701820174

[73] Smith TB, Rodríguez MD, Bernal G. Culture. Journal of Clinical Psychology. 2010;**67**(2):166-175. DOI: 10.1002/jclp.20757

[74] Smith TB, Trimble JE. Foundations of Multicultural Psychology: Research to Inform Effective Practice. Washington, DC: American Psychological Association; 2016

[75] Loon AV, Schaik AV, Dekker J, Beekman A. Bridging the gap for ethnic minority adult outpatients with depression and anxiety disorders by culturally adapted treatments. Journal of Affective Disorders. 2013;**147**(1-3): 9-16. DOI: 10.1016/j.jad.2012.12.014

[76] Ulibarri M, Calzada E, Cervantes RC, Santisteban DS, Bernal G. Make Your program work: The value of cultural adaptations for Latino-serving substance use treatment organizations. In: National Hispanic and Latino Addiction Technology Transfer Center ATTC. Los Angeles, CA; 2018

Section 3

Treatment

Chapter 3

A Spirituality Discourse in Treating Substance Use Disorders with Marginalised Persons

Shernaaz Carelse

Abstract

A spirituality discourse in substance abuse treatment offers useful unconventional constructs in treatment services to ethnic minority groups with substance use disorder (SUDs). It is important to locate spirituality within culture, place, and history in order to understand the spiritual needs of persons from minority groups with SUDs. There are many studies that merit a spiritual approach in treatment for ethnic minority groups with SUDs. However, spirituality is a broad concept that means different things to different people. Therefore, such an unconventional approach should be approached critically and cautiously. This chapter looks at the utilisation of an integrated eclectic approach with a focus on inclusion of spirituality in treatment services from a biopsychosocial-spiritual perspective. Tapping into the spiritual needs and the meaning that people ascribe to spirituality and religion (S&R) in treatment services is often more valued than conventional secular treatment services. Also, the client's spirituality is generally overlooked by professionals offering such services simply because it is so controversial. This chapter proposes an integrated eclectic methodology calling for a biopsychosocial-spiritual perspective to address the needs and well-being of ethnic minority groups with SUDs as a comprehensive person-centred and holistic approach, utilising mindfulness techniques.

Keywords: biopsychosocial-spiritual perspective, integrated electric methodology, mindfulness, person-centred, spirituality discourse, spirituality and religion, substance use disorder

1. Introduction

Similar to international trends, substance abuse is a huge concern and growing phenomenon in South Africa. Similarly more and more persons seeking treatment for substance use disorders (SUDs) present with dual diagnoses of which mental health problems are significantly high [1]. Treatment for SUDs thus has become more complex in that diagnoses and expectations of clients are multifaceted [1, 2]. Equally complex is treating clients with SUDs while paying due diligence to their ethnic, cultural and religious orientation. This chapter presents examples from a research study conducted in South Africa that supports the urgency for an integrated approach that incorporates spirituality in treating coloured persons with SUDs. It needs to point out that coloured people are not part of a minority group as described in conventional terms. However, they are marginalised and at a disadvantage in terms of their low socioeconomic status largely due to the remnants of apartheid,[1] laws in which the wealth and resources of the country were qualitatively and quantitatively unequally distributed to benefit a minority group in the country at the time [5]. The narratives that will be shared in this chapter are that of persons whose families were forcefully removed from urbanised towns to the outskirts of these towns to areas known as townships in terms of the then South African Group Areas Act of 1950 [3, 4]. While these township communities were characterised by social cohesion and a spirit of Ubuntu[2] [6], often still prevalent today, there were high crime rates and excessive use of alcohol and other drugs (AOD).

Today, 25 years after apartheid has been abolished in South Africa, townships continue to be plagued by poverty, unemployment and a high prevalence of SUDs [4, 7, 8]. As such treatment services offered by community-based non-profit organisations (NPOs) to coloured persons with SUDs are complex firstly, because people have deep psychosocial problems (such as previous disadvantage and high prevalence of poverty), and secondly, these township communities lack resources, such as clinics and hospitals that are overcrowded). Adding to these challenges is the fact that social workers rarely delve into the spiritual and religious (S&R) needs and well-being of clients leaving a gap in addressing the holistic needs of clients [8]. However, there is a growing body of literature that supports working with clients' spirituality, as an effective strategy in treating SUDs [8–13]. The literature also indicates an acknowledgement to facilitate ethnic minority groups' need for inclusion of their spirituality in treating SUDs [8, 14–16]. Such an approach calls for a broader perspective that pays equal attention to the biological, psychological, social and spiritual needs of people with SUDs. Furthermore one cannot look at such an integrated approach without considering mindfulness techniques which is an integral part of such spiritual conventions. It is against this backdrop that this chapter is presented.

2. An integrated eclectic approach for treating SUDs

There is no singular practice model in social work and/or SUD treatment that can be applied in all contexts. As such the intervention model that counsellors, such as social workers, select is unique to the setting and client often culminating in an eclectic approach [17]. Eclecticism is commonly used in social work and SUD treatment. It is the use of a wide range of theories and techniques regardless of its theoretical origins and orientation as long as the client, a group or a community's needs are met [18, 19]. In other words a social worker drawing on eclectic knowledge therefore uses a wide range of theories and techniques that are appropriate for a particular case. Similarly, an integrated approach is also the use of a combination of theories and techniques to address complex needs of individuals, groups and communities. The difference is that eclecticism does not necessarily result in the emergence of a new theory or model, while this is certainly the case with an integrated approach [18, 20].

There are approximately 400 new approaches that have evolved as a result of the integrationist movement, referred to as 'an ubiquitous process of conjunction that comes from relationship and conflict' [20]. Two perspectives that are important to understanding an integrated approach are chaos and complexity science and contiguous integration. Chaos and complexity science is driven by relational

---

[1] Apartheid was institutionalised laws and policies by the National Party in South Africa in 1945 which instituted policy and legislation that separated people on the basis of skin colour during 1945–1994 [3, 4].

[2] Ubuntu is a Zulu word that refers to humanity of an individual and/or society and principles of respect for the worth, dignity and humanity of self and others [6].

dynamics and systems theory, while contiguous integration holds that a person is understood in relation to larger groups, organisations or society, a perspective based on a metasystem view of the integration phenomenon [20]. This phenomenon is similar to the concept of Ubuntu in South Africa that holds that a person's worth and dignity is engrained and embedded in relation to others; therefore the saying in Ubuntu: 'I am because you are' [6].

The term integrated approach seems to have replaced the term eclectic approach [18, 19]. However, the two should not be confused and used interchangeably because it means different things. While an eclectic approach is more focused on the techniques used, an integrated approach focused on the theories and techniques and the emergence of a new theory [18]. There is, however, 'no technical eclectic that can totally disregard theory and no theoretical integrationist can totally ignore technique' [18, 20]. For example, social workers often use a biopsychosocial approach to treating SUDs. When social workers are confronted by clients to integrate clients' S&R, social workers are required to explore clients' S&R. Hence a fourth dimension, namely, spirituality, is necessary in an existing model or approach such as in a biopsychosocial model. This would involve not only knowledge of diverse S&R but also interrogating one's own S&R as a therapist.

It is appropriate to link what has been said thus far to the integrated relational model which places emphasis on the relationship of the client/patient and counsellor/doctor. Clients' response to treatment is the best indicator of treatment outcomes. An empathic counsellor/doctor improves and enhances treatment outcomes [21] especially when a strengths-based and problem-solving approach is adopted [22]. The integrated relational approach combines and has several principles in common with patient-centred, person-centred and problem-solving approaches.

A patient-centred approach is a commonly used approach in health settings and takes into consideration the patient's choices and decisions for accepting or declining medical care or procedures [23, 24]. Often a patient's S&R determines and affects his/her choices and decisions for medical intervention. Patient-centredness is often used interchangeably with person-centredness; however, the two are different [24, 25]. Similar to the patient-centred approach, this approach places the focus of intervention on developing relationships and care plans based on the client's preference [24, 26, 27]. However, a person-centred approach goes further and takes into consideration the ethical and legal rights of clients as important factors when providing holistic service [27]. A person-centred approach is therefore more holistic than a patient-centred approach [28]. Adding to the two aforementioned approaches is the problem-solving approach which is a generalist approach in social work that consists of distinct steps for effective problem-solving ([27, 28] Mc **and** Mc 2015). In short, the steps that a social worker will follow are: (1) Determining the exact nature of the problem—If the problem seems too complex, break it up into smaller manageable parts that can be managed one at a time. (2) Finding as many solutions to the problem as possible—Ask for input from clients and colleagues. (3) Narrowing down solutions—Anticipate possible outcomes of each choice, both negative and positive, and list anticipated consequences. (4) Making decision—Mutually decide with the client on what do. (5) Implementing the plan—Be cognizant of the outcome and use the success and challenges to improve and reassess the intervention goals [17]. The three approaches share similar principles worth exploring when working with persons having SUDs.

The common principles in the three approaches are summed up in **Table 1** as follows:

Table 1 presents the principles embedded in patient-centred [24, 25], person-centred [27, 28] and problem-solving [17] approaches. For the purpose of this chapter and since references to persons with SUDs do not only refer to such persons in

Client	The 'expert' in his/her own life		Has the freedom to make his/her own choices	
Counsellor	• Respects the client's worldview • Regards clients as the 'expert' in their own lives	• Emphasises clients' strengths • Views client as capable and motivated to move to wellness	• Responsible to meet clients where they are at • Fosters a therapeutic relationship that would facilitate opportunity for clients to take the responsibility for change	• Gives clients the freedom to make their own choices • Works within clients' frame of reference
Professional relationship	Fundamental to the therapeutic progress	Cooperation rather than confrontation	Goals and expectations for treatment are clearly articulated	

Table 1.
Principles of patient-centred, person-centred and problem-solving approaches.

medical or health settings but also in community-based settings, I will use the terms client (as in service user) and worker (as in service provider) whether in health or community-based setting. The client-worker relationship forms the foundation of the treatment process [17, 24, 27, 28]. The responsibilities and commitment of the worker is the second layer in the treatment process because an emphatic worker encourages clients' motivation for change. The last layer is the clients' role and responsibility as the 'expert' in his/her own life. The principles are not static but interlinked and fluid. The similarities of the principles in these approaches compliment an integrated eclectic model. While the principles may not specifically address spirituality per say, the inference to respect for the client's worldview, beginning where the client is at, honing in on the client's strengths and working in the client's frame of reference could be linked to clients' S&R.

2.1 Biopsychosocial model for treating SUDs

Originally developed for the medical sciences, George Engel (1933–1999) first introduced the biopsychosocial model in the health sciences. Engel [23] laid the foundation for a biopsychosocial model in healthcare. He argued that there is a distinctive interaction between the biological, psychological and social needs of patients that determine the cause, effects and outcomes of disease and well-being [23].

The concept of biopsychosocial model is eloquently described by Borrell-Carrió et al. [29] who propose that the model is a philosophy of clinical care and a practical guide for health practitioners. These authors argue that the model is philosophical on the one hand because it is a means of understanding how multiple levels of organisation, from the societal to the molecular, affect disease, illness and suffering. They further contend that the biopsychosocial model is practical in that it is a way of understanding the patient's subjective experience as an essential contributing factor to accurate diagnosis, health and humane care [29]. White, Williams and Greenberg [30] took this approach even further by introducing an ecological model of care that added the person in his/her environment context. White et al.'s model thus proposes that the biological, psychological and interpersonal relationships that surround a person require equal attention to achieve a state of health and well-being [30]. The two models, however, did not address the person's spirituality.

The addition of a spiritual dimension to define health was tabled at the 52nd Assembly of the World Health Organization (WHO). The 1948 WHO definition is 'Health is a state of complete physical, mental and social well-being, and not merely the absence of disease or infirmity'. Thus the proposed definition would be: 'Health is a dynamic state of complete physical, mental, spiritual and social well-being and not merely the absence of disease or infirmity'. Despite the latter being approved at the 1999, the 52nd WHO Assembly, it was not implemented [30]. Katerndahl [12] and Sulmasy, [31] while in favour of the spiritual dimension to the biopsychosocial model, however, warn that spirituality is a complex phenomenon and therefore should be approached critically when practitioners adopt a biopsychosocial-spiritual model in any context.

2.1.1 Biopsychosocial-spiritual model for treating SUDs

In the current milieu of treating ethnic minorities with SUDs, the reductionist scientific model is inadequate to meet the holistic needs of clients [32]. Therefore, a biopsychosocial-spiritual model for treating ethnic minorities with SUDs which utilises mindfulness techniques is proposed. Mindfulness approaches in treating persons with mental health and related conditions are rooted in Buddhist Vipassana meditation, which was introduced by Kabat-Zinn in 1979 [33]. Mindfulness approaches involves 'paying attention in a particular way; on purpose in the present moment' in a non-judgemental way [34, 35]. It involves being aware of and accepting of thoughts and acknowledging and accepting livid experiences, thoughts and feelings instead of modifying and/or suppressing such experiences, thoughts and feelings [35]. In other words clients are encouraged to practise 'reperceiving' (think of SUD, e.g. differently, as an issue externalised rather than internalised) and 'attentional control' (how to externalised SUD) which could facilitate a more mindful response to SUD [33]. So, mindfulness is the practice and process of beginning where the client is at, being cognizant of the 'here and now' and 'being in the present moment' [33–36]. Furthermore, focusing on the here and now could help the client to enhance and improve focus, have a greater awareness and gain perspective regarding the SUD and the adverse consequences associated with it. Using mindfulness techniques could assist the client in recognising risks associated with relapse and could thus assist in avoiding relapse [36]. Skills to facilitate mindfulness techniques can be taught to diverse people regardless of cultural S&R backgrounds and can be used in a variety of intervention approaches such as biopsychosocial-spiritual models [34, 35, 37].

While the need for a biopsychosocial-spiritual model utilising mindfulness techniques in SUDs has been well established [34–37], it is not clear how this new model can be integrated within the reductionist scientific conception of the client. Several empirical studies and systematic literature reviews [9, 20, 29, 31] are drawn on explaining how a biopsychosocial-spiritual model for treatment in SUDs is worth perusing as a feasible approach for working with ethnic minorities. But first it is imperative to explain the distinction between spirituality and religion.

2.1.1.1 Spirituality and religion

Spirituality and religion (S&R) is often used interchangeably as if it means the same thing. What is more, there is not a universal definition for either mainly because the two respective constructs are so diverse [8, 38–40]. S&R has to do with one's beliefs, emotional state of mind experiences and conduct associated with the search for the sacred [10, 39]. At the same time, it can be described as a worldview that places emphasis on the divine, a higher power or being whose followers promote

Spirituality	Religion
• A holistic approach • Captures diverse cultures and beliefs • Ascribe meaning, purpose and morality • Creates awareness of social obligations and relations with self, others, the universe and reality • Facilitates engagement with other dimensions of the universe such as divinity, with God and/or other beings	• An organised set of beliefs • A system of beliefs and practices that is shared by a community of people • Comprises rules and rituals to be observed • Rituals offered and communicated to the divine, sacred, God • Rules and rituals are institutionalised

Table 2.
Spirituality vs. religion.

spiritual and human well-being in which care and compassion for others take a centre stage as apposed to self-centred materialistic gains [13, 39, 41]. In this chapter, however, briefly, I differentiate between spirituality and religion (see **Table 2**).

In reference to **Table 2**, religion for most part is about a set of beliefs about the moral code governing human conduct, while spirituality is not constrained by theological barriers and/or any particular ideology [38]. Rather it is characterised as the quest to understand and find answers to definitive questions about life, about meaning and about relationship to the divine, sacred or God and may (or may not) emanate from or lead to the development of religious rituals and rules [39]. Spirituality is thus a more holistic and inclusive approach as apposed to religion. Spirituality is rooted in multiculturalism and is therefore diverse in terms of cultures and beliefs [38]. The search for meaning, purpose and morality and fulfilling relations with self, others, the universe and ultimately with reality are central to spirituality [40, 41]. Ubuntu shares similar principles. Spirituality (however a person understands it) has always been part of indigenous and culturally sensitive substance abuse counselling [29]; consider, for example, Alcoholics Anonymous (AA) programmes. I propose that the spiritual dimension (which includes religiosity) should be recognised and incorporated in treatment models regardless of the field of practice.

2.1.1.2 Understanding the spiritual needs of people with SUDs

> *"What treatment, by whom, is more effective for this individual with that specific problem and under which set of circumstances?" [42]*

Social workers treating ethnic minorities with SUDs are confronted with complex challenges experienced by clients. Never has Paul's [42] provocative question been more valid than in the current milieu of SUDs. Understanding the spiritual needs of persons with SUD is important if we are truly holistic in our approach to service delivery and should thus not be perceived as separate from attending to biopsychosocial needs. To holistically assess people with complex challenges associated with SUDs, knowledge about their spirituality is important [43–45] and can thus not be avoided, especially when client themselves raise the need to delve into their S&R.

Several qualitative studies [14, 38, 40, 43, 44, 46] that investigated religious coping and spirituality in relation to SUDs indicate that positive religious coping and dimensions of spirituality protect against SUDs. In a qualitative study [47] that focused on barriers and facilitators to successful transition from long-term residential substance abuse treatment, the researchers found that clients having faith in the

Divine as a facilitator for transitioning from in-patient treatment to reintegration back into the family and community played a pivotal role during the reintegration process. Various studies [8, 45–48] indicate the value of addressing S&R as a factor that enhances and aids treatment for SUDs. However, several studies with ethnic minorities [8, 46, 48, 49] have found that the S&R needs of clients are not generally addressed by counsellors (such as social workers), and instead this role is more likely to be facilitated by clergy and/or recovering addicts. This raises the question though: who should be facilitating this role if clients make explicit their need for S&R well-being? If such high value is placed on the S&R of clients, a counsellor will require some understanding of S&R albeit at a theoretical level in order to effectively provide treatment services. It stands to reason therefore that a biopsychosocial-spiritual approach requires the counsellor to reflect and interrogate his/her own S&R as well as his/her own ambivalence for not wanting to venture into clients' S&R.

3. A spiritual dimension in treating SUDs

Employing a spiritual dimension in treating SUDs is not a new phenomenon. The complexity of dual diagnoses and the multifaceted challenges associated with SUDs necessitated a need to intervene beyond the biological, psychological and social needs of clients with SUDs [1, 2, 8, 10, 15].

3.1 Spirituality and religious coping

South Africans are not averse to managing complex life challenges through prayer, meditation and rituals as coping measures. Such practices are often embedded in people's spirituality which is commonly rooted in their religion and/or culture [6, 9, 16]. The reflections shared next is that of participants in a recent qualitative research study conducted in the Western Cape of South Africa on the experiences of coloured adults seeking substance abuse services at non-profit organisations (NPOs) [8].

John[*3], 32, has been in and out of rehab since he was 14 years old. Most of the rehabs he has been to in the past were what he refers to as *secular* rehabs, meaning that it did not have a spiritual component in its treatment model. According to the facility manager, this is the longest that John has been sober and attributes this to the fact that John is in a faith-based rehab that employs a biopsychosocial-spiritual model. This is John's narrative of his experience of S&R coping:

> *I started using when I was very young, I must have been like fourteen years old. I went to an organisation that was an out-patient programme where they basically counseled me on a weekly basis. This time is different because there is a strong focus on the spiritual side of the addict. Because of my religious background I am more at home at this rehab and I know if I keep to the programme I will stay sober.*

John's situation is indeed complex as SUD cases generally are. Apart from the SUD, he experienced marital problems and homelessness, and his estranged wife refused to grant him visitations with their children. The complexity of SUDs often leaves people discouraged, and many, such as in the case of John, acknowledged drawing strength from God, a higher power, and being part of a religious group that meets on a weekly basis [49]. Like many people with SUDs, John felt that delving into S&R of clients provides a more holistic treatment approach than secular approaches that avoid S&R completely [49–52].

[3] *Not the service users' real names

3.2 Spiritual mindfulness

While mindfulness theories originate from Buddhism, people of different religious affiliations have become more open to use these techniques because of its usefulness especially in treating SUDs. The use of meditation is a common practice in mindfulness techniques [34, 35, 37, 48]. A case example of a client with dual diagnoses explains the use of prayer as a form of mindfulness technique.

James*, 26, admits being addicted to drugs and sex. He says the sex craving started when he was rehabilitated and during his first treatment programme completion. He believed that when he gave up methamphetamine, the craving for smoking cigarettes started. While in the programme which was an in-patient treatment programme for adults with SUDs, James gave up cigarettes and methamphetamine. However, when he reintegrated back into his community, his cravings for sex started, something according to him that was never an issue in his life before being treated for SUDs. He related that he started smoking after having sex and then later reverted back to using methamphetamine to the point where he felt that he could not cope without using methamphetamine on a daily basis. He explained that he felt that his cravings for methamphetamine were worse than before because he failed God in falling back into drugs. He explains: 'The righteous will fall seven times...' which is a Bible first quoted from Proverbs 24:16–18. Making reference to the quoted scripture, he explained his relapse as follows:

> *...I didn't believe at first but I have experienced it firsthand. I was worse off in a space of a few months after beating my addiction to meth. ... I first started stealing. I sold my personal belongings. In a space of a few months I lost so much weight. I knew where it was going to end, because my mind was constantly on how to get my next fix. My family did not confront me, but they could clearly see that I was back on drugs again. I told my sister that the addiction was out of my control and that I wanted to go back to the rehab.*

James was reflecting and had a greater sense of spiritual mindfulness regarding the SUD and relapse because he described himself as follows:

> *I am a child of God, but I didn't work on all aspects of my life. I had to work on it [referring to his spiritual life]. So I did not equip myself adequately with the word [referring to the Bible] of God. So I am back [at the rehab] to work on a view aspects that I neglected before. So I can give people advice and can share the word of God to the people in my community. I can also refer them to a place for rehabilitation if they want help. But the best thing is to proclaim the Word of the Lord. You do not need a [rehabilitation] program. You can change your life just by adhering to the Word of God. It is easier said than done, but it can be done.*

James attributes his recovery to his spiritual awakening more than the intervention by social workers.

It is not uncommon that the need for close relationships with others and/or an encounter with a divine being or higher power is a motivating factor for maintained sobriety in people with SUDs [53]. Whatever the client's reason for wanting to maintain sobriety, the social worker should tap into the motivating factors and amplify it as strengths [54, 55]. Motivation is a state of readiness to change in which a predictable course is followed. This is where client-centred approaches such as motivational interviewing (MI) and motivational enhancement therapy (MET) are appropriate models because it is aimed at bringing about and enhancing change in the problem situation. These methods emphasise resolving clients' ambivalence [54, 55]. Honing in on client's motivating factors such as restoring relationships with significant others is important in enhancing motivation and resolving ambivalence. When clients are treated as partners, they are more likely to respond to the counsellor.

MI and MET do not represent any particular theoretical perspective and are thus useful to contextualise in terms of an integrated eclectic approach. Furthermore MI and MET are brief treatment strategies that can be as short as four sessions but can be prolonged depending on the client's level of motivation [53–55]. Thus intervention is time limited and goal directed, when the client reaches a level of high motivation where he/she is able to take responsibility for his/her own recovery.

3.3 Spirituality as a component in treatment programmes

Many community-based organisations in South Africa offer a dual focus, meaning the treatment service includes both a secular social work intervention approach and a spiritual approach. However, the spiritual component is mostly offered by volunteers who are religious leaders in the communities where the organisations are situated. During the course of the day, most of the programmes make provision for meditation and prayer. So clients gather in groups in separate venues or those who preferred to meditate on their own would find a private space in the organisation to engage in prayer and meditation [8].

Strategies employed in self-help groups [56, 57] that focus on the cognitive, spiritual and behaviour changes of the persons with SUDs are more accessible because they are found across communities and are free of charge [52]. However, organisations should caution against whom and what such rituals entail so as not to exploit and/or impose religion or spirituality on clients. Therefore general training should be available for all people involved in substance abuse services including volunteers. It is imperative for such persons to have basic standards and knowledge for practice to avoid possible harm to clients. With the review and implementation of the current White Paper on Health (NHI) [58] and the norms and standards for social welfare services in South Africa, this type and methods of interventions are worth pursuing as services become more expensive and therefore inaccessible to the clients who come from disadvantaged communities, are unemployed and have low incomes.

3.4 Spirituality of the counsellor

Social worker rarely set out to gage clients about their spirituality. However, this topic more often than not emerges during interviews and thus requires social workers to be knowledgeable not necessarily on every spiritual and/or religious practice out there, but at least being able to engage client's expression of his/her S&R needs [59, 60]. This unconventional way of looking at treating SUDs is particularly important in the South African context, where spirituality is ingrained in the culture and value systems of many South Africans and more so in the light of current policy and legislation in South Africa calling for evidence-based, culturally sensitive and indigenous practice and research [8]. As counsellors treating ethnic minorities with SUDs, social workers are encouraged to interrogate their own spirituality, as clients more often than not express their own spiritual needs during treatment services [61, 62].

It is not uncommon that group work offered by NPOs is generally facilitated by laypersons such as spiritual counsellors [8, 63, 64]. In some instances these would be trained clergy [63]; however, in most cases these would be recovering addicts [8, 51, 57] who have had some 'supernatural' experience. This is similar to approaches used in self-help groups such as Alcoholics Anonymous. The focus of such programmes is that most of the group work interventions are on spiritual growth and life skills [8, 65]. For example, in a study conducted by carelse [8] that focused on ethnic minority groups in treatment for methamphetamine, all the participants reported on the important role played by religious clergy and recovering addicts. This is what they had to say:

> *We have two spiritual counsellors ...They focus more on the spiritual things like the Christian principles.*
>
> *And then we have a lot of ministers and pastors, and ... priests, since the organisation is a faith-based organisation. We do spiritual growth which is run by pastors.*

These narratives concur with studies conducted [50, 57, 63] that focused on professionals and laypersons' contention with issues of power, oppression and privilege in service delivery. These authors conclude that there must be differentiating functions of professionals such as social workers and laypersons such as recovering addicts in the helping relationship. As a general rule, training should be available for all people involved in services to people with SUDs including volunteers, in particular training on how to engage the service user's spirituality [60, 61]. Therefore it is imperative for clergy and recovering addicts in treatment in SUDs to have basic standards and knowledge with regard to spiritual intervention to avoid possible harm to clients. More importantly service providers will have to interrogate their own spirituality (however they perceive it) in order to engage meaningfully with the spirituality of others.

3.5 Spirituality and maintained sobriety

In pursuing a state of equilibrium, clients feel that it was important for them to take the first step of the 12-step programme [57, 62] and admit that they were powerless over SUDs and that their lives had become unmanageable. In particular, clients in the 12-step programmes believed that a power greater than themselves could restore their emotional and spiritual well-being [62] where spirituality and a connection to a higher power are pivotal to their recovery process. These are some of their perspectives in this regard from a study on the coping resources of a minority group of adults in a low socioeconomic community on the outskirts of Cape Town, South Africa [8]:

> *It brought me closer to my higher father and relying on him and to acknowledge that he took me out of, how can I say, I was lost totally.*
>
> *I believe it's prayer that God is opening for me. And I never prayed when I was using ... my mind was all over the place but now I pray with sincerity and without any mind-altering.*

The clients' livid experiences are confirmed in the study by Miller and Rollnick [55] that explored the role of spirituality in the intervention outcomes after a 12-step programme. As Miller and Rollnick [55] points out, clients experienced an increased spiritual awareness and growth after completing the treatment programme. The findings also suggest that spirituality may have a positive effect on maintained sobriety if the person continues to engage in mindfulness strategies. In a study by Amaro and Black on the role of spirituality in helping Black women with histories of trauma and substance abuse, healing and recovery of participants also expressed more hope and motivation to maintain their sobriety because of their spiritual awareness and growth after their involvement in a programme incorporating mindfulness strategies linked to spirituality during treatment [35].

3.6 Spiritual complementary therapies

Treatment services for SUDs sometimes involve alternative therapies too [34, 37, 62]. For ethnic minorities in low socioeconomic community, alternative therapies such as reflexology are not common [8]. Participants could experience being overwhelmed with such unfamiliar strategies as one client indicated [8]: 'I could not believe that someone so decent touched me. Me, I am an addict. People normally treat us as dirty and filth, the low lives of society'. Therefore clients must be introduced to such new methods in a client-centred manner that respects their S&R and cultural believes.

The social worker's personal religiosity, training and sensitivity to the client's spirituality help in using an integrative approach that includes clients' alternative therapies [10, 20, 23, 64]. Therefore, educating and sensitising social workers in terms of S&R and alternative therapies are of paramount importance [23, 40, 44, 50, 55, 63, 65]. Ongoing training and intrinsic spirituality on the part of the social worker offering services to people with SUDs could be a catalyst when using an integrated approach [60, 63–65].

There is a growing body of literature on spiritual complementary or alternative therapies; however, there is a dearth of research of its efficacy for treating ethnic minorities with SUDs [?]. Still, an integrated body, mind and spirit approach to intervention in social work practice that is researched- and therefore evidence-based can be an advantage in treating such groups [62]. A combination of Eastern and Western philosophies as well as current research in integrated practice approach offering guidelines for assessment and intervention and not limited to spiritual beliefs appears to be a viable approach.

3.7 Spirituality as a foundation for restoring human dignity

The role of the social worker in any setting is to provide support and guidance. Participants in Carelse's study [8] reported that the counselling, interest and compassion from the social workers motivated them to stay in the programme and to pursue their recovery goals. They described the service provided as very good work, noting that all the things they had learnt would help to prevent relapse, to stay positive and to keep their focus on their recovery goals. Participants' views about the benefits of utilising social work services provided by the NPOs offering treatment to adults with SUDs from low socioeconomic backgrounds are summed up as follows:

> *The drugs strip you of all that [dignity] and I think that's a big part of a social worker's duty in individual counselling. They do very good work and even after I finished [the drug counselling programme] the one lady called and she wasn't even my therapist, and she called and followed up. She called to my mom's because she couldn't get a hold of me, how am I doing and that. And at that time, I relapsed already so I felt guilty ... So that for me played a big role, the interest. And I think that's a major role; the compassion with which you do your work.*

> *All the things you learn there and the chance to express yourself. The information is vital, what they [social workers] put in place, a plan to prevent relapse and I still have all my papers [literature/material on coping resources] at home. And the homework that they give you, it keeps you positive, it keeps you focused on your goal to stay clean. So that helps a lot.*

> *I started praying again. I prayed Wednesday and Thursday and felt better spiritually. Even though I'm not on the place, I know I won't fool myself to think that now that I am praying I am recovered. Friday a lady called me and said she's got a job*

> *for me so everything is coming together. So things are starting to fall in place for me and I believe its prayer that God is opening doors for me.*

> *I never prayed when I was using, because I was constantly under the influence [of drugs] and I felt unworthy. Not that I feel worthy now but at least I now don't have drugs in my system. My mind is all over the place but I pray to make myself feel better. Now I pray with sincerity and without any mind-altering [drugs].*

The benefits of prayer and meditation seem to have developed the client's problem-solving techniques and efforts to manage triggers for relapse. Coping with stress and stressors such as in the case of SUDs involves deliberate efforts such as in mindfulness strategies, which in this study were prayer and meditation to combat and deter SUDs by influencing the environment and using the resources such as mindfulness strategies in the form of prayer and meditation [34, 35, 37, 62]. Therefore it can be deduced that maintained sobriety is largely dependent on the nature and scope of the treatment programme and more so when mindfulness strategies in a biopsychosocial-spiritual approach is embedded in treatment. Incorporating spirituality in the treatment programmes challenges clients to reflect on their quality of life, for example, learning new ways of dealing with SUDs enhances their self-worth and dignity as they gain higher levels of person: environment fit or a state of equilibrium.

4. Conclusion

There is a growing demand for integrated approaches to treating minority and marginalised people with SUDs. Such treatment requires a continuous process of interrogating theories and related approaches to suit clients' needs. Social work services have evolved from a generalist approach to a person-centred approach over the past 20 years. In this process, the spiritual dimension to persons with SUDs gained progressively more prominence. Currently, a biopsychosocial-spiritual approach has paramount importance for offering integrated and holistic treatment for ethnic minority persons with SUDs. Thus a biopsychosocial-spiritual approach is proposed particularly in the South African context where spirituality is ingrained in the culture and value systems of coloured people. This chapter highlighted the importance of an integrated eclectic approach and the feasibility of a biopsychosocial-spiritual model in treating SUDs in marginalised communities in South Africa. Lessons could be learnt from the experiences shared for integrating spirituality in SUDs in similar contexts. What is clear is that the value of a biopsychosocial-spiritual approach in substance abuse treatment in South Africa cannot be ignored. By no means, this is the only model that can be used with marginalised communities, but it is one that is emerging strongly in treating SUDs when working with such ethnic minorities. The value of spirituality as it relates to person-centredness, in treating SUDs in minority groups, is a topic worth pursuing for future research.

The inclusion of a person-centred approach and mindfulness strategies in treating SUDs should also be further investigated. Similarly, the Bachelor of Social Work (BSW) as well as continued professional development training should incorporate aspects of students' and practitioners' personal spiritual beliefs, the role this has on the professional relationship, as well as the impact of spirituality on the intervention process. Therefore it will be imperative that due diligence is given to the personal S&R beliefs (whether they believe in the transcendent, a higher power or not) of students and practitioners because it is as important as that of the clients that they serve.

The biopsychosocial-spiritual model is indeed a modern humanistic and holistic perspective that is truly person-centred and therefore worth perusing for treatment services with marginalised persons with SUDs, such as ethnic minorities.

Conflict of interest

The author declares no conflict of interest.

Author details

Shernaaz Carelse
University of the Western Cape, Cape Town, South Africa

*Address all correspondence to: scarelse@uwc.ac.za

References

[1] South African Community Epidemiology Network on Drug Abuse. Research Brief. Medical Research Council. [Internet]. 2017. Available from: http://www.mrc.ac.za/adarg/sacendu.htm [Accessed: 2017/08/12]

[2] Crisp C. Dual diagnosis: Substance abuse and mental health in an inpatient setting. In: Grobman LM, editor. Days in the Lives of Social Workers. 3rd ed. Harrisburg, PA: White Hat Communications; 2005. pp. 205-210. ISBN: 10: 0965365387

[3] South African History [Internet]. A history of Apartheid in South Africa. Available: https://www.sahistory.org.za/article/history-apartheid-south-africa [Accessed: 2019/07/16]

[4] Kirk JF. Making a Voice: African Resistance to Segregation in South Africa. 1st ed. New York: Routledge; 2018. 368 p 9780429499104

[5] Patel L. Social Welfare and Social Development. 2nd ed. Cape Town: Oxford University Press; 2015. 352 p

[6] Mangena F. African ethics through Ubuntu: A postmodern exposition. Africology: The Journal of Pan African Studies. 2016;**2**:66-80. Available from: http://www.jpanafrican.org/docs/vol9no2/9.2-6-Fainos.pdf [Accessed: 2019/07/20]

[7] De Lannoy A. Unpacking the Lived Realities of Western Cape Youth. Exploring the well-being of young people residing in five of the most deprived areas in the Western Cape Province. Available from: www.povertyandinequality.uct.ac.za/sites/default/files/image_tool/images/95/2018/Publications/Youth%20Well%20being%20WC_Research-report.pdf [Accessed: 2018/07/20]

[8] Carelse S. Social Work Services Provided by Non-profit Organisations to Adult Methamphetamine Uses – An Ecological Systems Perspective [Thesis]. Stellenbosch: Stellenbosch University; 2018

[9] Dreyer Y. Community resilience and spirituality: Keys to hope for a post-apartheid South Africa. Pastoral Psychology. 2015;**64**:651-662. DOI: 10.1007/s11089-014-0632-2

[10] Philips C. Spirituality in social work: Introducing a spiritual dimension into social work education and practice. Social Work Research. 2014;**26**:65-77. DOI: 10.11157/anzswj-vol26iss4id27

[11] Ruglass LM, Yali AM. Do race/ethnicity and religious affiliation moderate treatment outcomes among individuals with co-occurring PTSD and substance use disorders? Journal of Prevention & Intervention in the Community. 2019;**47**(3):198-213. DOI: 10.1080/10852352.2019.1603674

[12] Katerndahl DA. Impact of spiritual symptoms and their interactions on health services and life satisfaction. Annals of Family Medicine. 2008;**6**: 412-420. DOI: 10.1370/afm.886

[13] Hutchison W. The role of religious auspiced agencies in the post-modern era. In: Meinert R, Pardeck J, Murphy J, editors. Postmodernism Religion and the Future of Social Work. Vol. 18. New York: The Haworth Press; 1998. pp. 55-69. DOI: 10.1080/15426432.1998.9960236

[14] Limb G, Hodge D. Developing spiritual lifemaps as a culture-centred pictorial instrument for spiritual assessments with native American clients. Research on Social Work Practice. 2007;**17**(2):296-304. DOI: 10.1177/1049731506296161

[15] Blakey JM. The role of spirituality in helping African American women with histories of trauma and substance

abuse heal and recover. Social Work and Christianity. 2016;**43**:40-59. ISSN: 1944-7779

[16] Dykes G, Carelse S. Spirituality. In: Van Breda A, Sekudu J, editors. Theories for Decolonial Social Work Practice in South Africa. Cape Town, South Africa: Oxford University Press; 2019. ISBN: 9780190721350.ch12

[17] Coady N, Lehmann P, editors. Theoretical Perspectives for Direct Social Work Practice: A Generalist-Eclectic Approach. 3rd ed. New York: Springer Publishing Company; 2016 . 469 p. ISBN: 13-9780826119476

[18] Norcross JC, Grencavage LM. Eclecticism and integration in counseling and psychotherapy: Major themes and obstacles. In: Dryden W, Norcross JC, Grencavage LM. Eclecticism and integration in counselling and psychotherapy: Major themes and obstacle. British Journal of Guidance and Counselling. 1989;**17**:227-247. DOI: 10.1080/03069888908260036

[19] Nuttall J. Imperatives and perspectives of psychotherapy integration. International Journal of Psychotherapy. 2002;**7**:249-264. DOI: 10.1080/1356908021000063169

[20] Saad M, De Medeiros R, Mosini A. Opinion. Are we ready for a true biopsychosocial-spiritual model? The many meanings of 'spiritual'. Medicine. 2017;**4**:1-6. DOI: 10.3390/medicines4040079

[21] King DE. Faith, Spirituality and Medicine: Toward the Making of a Healing Practitioner. Binghamton, NY: Haworth Pastoral Press; 2000. ISBN: 13-978-0789011152

[22] McKee DD, Chappel JN. Spirituality and medical practice. Journal of Family Practice. 1992;**35**:201, 205-208. Available from: https://europepmc.org/abstract/med/1645114 [Accessed: 20/07/20]

[23] Engel GL. How much longer must medicine's science be bound by a seventeenth century world view? Psychotherapy and Psychosomatics. 1992;**57**:3-16. DOI: 10.1159/000288568

[24] Slater L. Person-centredness: A concept analysis. Contemporary Nurse. 2006;**23**(1):135-144. DOI: 10.5172/conu.2006.23.1.135

[25] Connor JP, Haber PS, Hall WD. Alcohol use disorders. The Lancet. 2016;**387**(10022):988-998. DOI: 10.1016/S0140-6736(15)00122-1

[26] McNeil R, Kerr T, Pauly B, Wood E, Small W. Advancing patient-centered care for structurally vulnerable drug-using populations: A qualitative study of the perspectives of people who use drugs regarding the potential integration of harm reduction interventions into hospitals. Addiction. 2016;**111**(4):685-694. DOI: 10.1111/add.13214

[27] Zhao J, Gao S, Wang J, Liu X, Hao Y. Differentiation between two healthcare concepts: Person-centered and patient-centered care. International Journal of Nursing Sciences. 2016;**3**(4):398-402

[28] McCance T, McCormack B. The person-centred practice framework. In: Person-Centred Practice in Nursing and Health Care: Theory and Practice. Chichester, West Sussex, UK; 2016. pp. 36-62. Chap 3. ISBN: 8781118990575

[29] Borrell-Carrió F, Suchman A, Epstein R. The biopsychosocial model 25 years later: Principles, practice, and scientific inquiry. Annals of Family Medicine. 2004;**6**:576-582. DOI: 10.1370/afm.245

[30] White KL, Williams TF, Greenberg BG. The ecology of medical care. Bulletin of the New York Academy of Medicine. 1996;**73**:187-212. Available

from: bullnyacadmed01031-0195.pdf [Accessed: 2019/07/20]

[31] Sulmasy DP. A biopsychosocial-spiritual model for the care of patients at the end of life. Gerontologist. 2002;**42**: 24-33. DOI: 10.1093/geront/42.suppl_3.24

[32] Smith RL, Southern S. Integrative confusion: An examination of integrative models in couple and family therapy. The Family Journal. 2014;**13**:392-399. Available from: http://tfj.sagepub.com/content/13/4/392 [Accessed: 2019/07/15]

[33] Marcus MT, Zgierska A. Mindfulness Related Treatment and Addiction Recovery. New York: Routledge; 2012, 2012. ISBN: 13: 978 0415 69689 0

[34] Li W, Howard MO, Garland EL, McGovern P, Lazar M. Mindfulness treatment for substance misuse: A systematic review and meta-analysis. Journal of Substance Abuse Treatment. 2017;**75**:62-96

[35] Amaro H, Black DS. Moment-by-moment in Women's recovery: Randomized controlled trial protocol to test the efficacy of a mindfulness-based intervention on treatment retention and relapse prevention among women in residential treatment for substance use disorder. Contemporary Clinical Trials. 2017;**62**:146-152. DOI: 10.1016/j.cct.2017.09.004

[36] Turner T, Welsches P, Conti S. Mindfulness-Based Sobriety-a clinician's Guide for Addiction Recovery Using Relapse Prevention Therapy, Acceptance & Commitment Therapy & Motivational Interviewing. Canada: Raincoast Books; 2013. ISBN: 978 160882 854 8

[37] Bautista T, James D, Amaro H. Acceptability of mindfulness-based interventions for substance use disorder: A systematic review. Complementary Therapies in Clinical Practice. 2019;**35**:201-207. DOI: 10.1016/j.ctcp.2019.02.012

[38] Holloway M, Moss B. Spirituality in Social Work. Basingstoke, Hampshire, UK: Palgrave McMillan; 2010. ISBN: 13 978 230 21924 3

[39] Koenig HG, King DE, Carson VB. Handbook of Religion and Health 2nd Ed. New York: Oxford University Press; 2012. 1192 p. ISBN: 9780195335958

[40] Furman L, Benson P, Grimwood C, Canda E. Religion and spirituality in social work education and practice at the millennium: A survey of UK social workers. British Journal of Social Work. 2004;**34**:767-792. Available from: http://www.jstor.org/stable/23720509 [Accesssed: 2019/07/20]

[41] Kissman K, Mauer L. East meets west: Therapeutic aspects of spirituality in health, mental health and addiction recovery. International Social Work. 2002;**45**:35-43. DOI: 10.1177/0020872802045001315

[42] Paul GL. Strategy of outcome research in psychotherapy. Journal of Consulting Psychology. 1967;**31**:109-119. DOI: 10.1037/h0024436

[43] Stansley MA, Bush AL, Camp ME, Jameson JP, Philips LL, Barber CR. Older adults' preferences for religion/spirituality in treatment for anxiety and depression. Aging and Mental Health. 2011;**15**(3):334-343. DOI: 10.1080/13607863.2010.519326

[44] Oxhandler HK, Pargament KI. Social work practitioners' integration of clients' religion and spirituality in practice: A literature review. Social Work. 2014;**59**:271-279. DOI: 10.1093/sw/swu018

[45] Giordano AL, Prosek EA, Stamman J, Callahan MM, Loseu S, Bevly CM, et al. Addressing trauma in substance abuse

treatment. Journal of Alcohol and Drug Education. 2016;**60**:55

[46] Heinz AJ, Disney ER, Epstein DH, Glezen LA, Clark PI, Preston KL. A focus-group study on spirituality and substance-user treatment. Substance Use & Misuse. 2010;**45**:134-153. DOI: 10.3109/10826080903035130

[47] Manuel JI, Yuan Y, Herman DB, Svikis DS, Nichols O, Palmer E, et al. Barriers and facilitators to successful transition from long-term residential substance abuse treatment. Journal of Substance Abuse Treatment. 2017;**74**: 16-22. DOI: 10.1016/j.jsat.2016.12.001

[48] Shorey RC, Gawrysiak MJ, Anderson S, Stuart GL. Dispositional mindfulness, spirituality, and substance use in predicting depressive symptoms in a treatment-seeking sample. Journal of Clinical Psychology. 2015;**71**:334-345. DOI: 10.1002/jclp.22139

[49] Nedelec JL, Richardson G, Silver IA. Religiousness, spirituality, and substance use: A genetically sensitive examination and critique. Journal of Drug Issues. 2017;**47**:340-355. DOI: 10.1177/0022042617693382

[50] Canda ER. Spiritual connections in social work: Boundary violations and transcendence. Journal of Religion & Spirituality in Social Work: Social Thought. 2008;**27**(1-2):25-33. DOI: 10.1080/15426430802113749

[51] Best D, Beckwith M, Haslam C, Alexander Haslam S, Jetten J, Mawson E, et al. Overcoming alcohol and other drug addiction as a process of social identity transition: The social identity model of recovery (SIMOR). Addiction Research & Theory. 2016;**24**(2):111-123. DOI: 10.3109/16066359.2015.1075980

[52] Alcoholics Anonymous [Internet]. Alcoholics Anonymous 12-Step Recovery Programme. Available from: http://www.recovery.org/topics/alcoholics-anonymous-12-step/ [Accessed: 2018/08/24]

[53] Gaine GS, La Guardia JG. The unique contributions of motivations to maintain a relationship and motivations toward relational activities to relationship well-being. Motivation and Emotion. 2009;**33**(2):184-202. DOI: 10.1007/s11031-009-9120-x

[54] Wagner CC, Ingersoll KS. Motivational Interviewing in Groups. New York: Guilford Press; 2012. 416 p. ISBN 9781462507924

[55] Miller WR, Rollnick S. Motivational Interviewing: Helping People to Change. 3rd ed. New York: Guilford Press; 2013. ISBN: 13 978-1609182274

[56] Hettema J, Steele J, Miller WR. Motivational interviewing. Annual Review of Clinical Psychology. 2005;**1**:91-111. DOI: 10.1146/annurev.clinpsy.1.102803.143833

[57] Ranes B, Johnson R, Nelson L, Slaymaker V. The role of spirituality in treatment outcomes following a residential 12-step programme. Alcoholism Treatment Quarterly. 2017;**35**:1, 16-33. DOI: 10.1080/07347324.2016.1257275

[58] White Paper on Health. National Health Institute. South Africa, Pretoria. 2017. Available from: https://www.gov.za/sites/default/files/gcis_document/201512/39506gon1230.pdf [Accessed: 2019/07/20].

[59] Carrington A. A spiritual approach to social work practice. In: Crisp BR, editor. Handbook of Religion, Spirituality and Social Work. London, UK: Routledge; 2017, 2017. DOI: 10.4324/9781315679853

[60] Hodge DR. Spiritual competence. In: Crisp BR, editor. Handbook of Religion, Spirituality and Social Work. 1st ed. London, UK: Routledge; 2017. 398 p. ISBN: 9781315679853

[61] Oxhandler HK, Giardina TD. Social workers' perceived barriers to and sources of support for integrating clients' religion and spirituality in practice. Social Work. 2017;**62**(4): 323-332. DOI: 10.1093/sw/swx036

[62] Lee MY, Leung PP. Integrative Body-Mind-Spirit Social Work: An Empirically Based Approach to Assessment and Treatment. New York, USA: Oxford University Press; 2018. ISBN: 97801 90458522

[63] Tan SY, Scalise ET. Lay Counselling, Revised and Updated: Equipping Christians for a Helping Ministry. Michigan: Harper Collins Christian Publishing; 2016. 410 p. ISBN-13: 978-0310524274

[64] Chatters LM, Taylor RJ, Woodward AT, Bohnert AS, Peterson TL, Perron BE. Differences between African Americans and non-Hispanic whites utilization of clergy for counseling with serious personal problems. Race and Social Problems. 2017;**9**(2):139-149. DOI: 10.1007/s12552-017-9207-z

[65] Ali OM. The imam and the mental health of Muslims: Learning from research with other clergy. Journal of Muslim Mental Health. 2016;**50**(1):46-61. DOI: 10.3998/jmmh.10381607.0010.106

Chapter 4

Effective Treatment of Opioid Use Disorder among African Americans

Daniel L. Howard

Abstract

The current opioid epidemic substantially affects African Americans given their historical rate of disparities in access to effective substance use disorder (SUD) treatment. Yet, there is limited information about factors that may improve access to effective opioid use disorder (OUD) treatment for members of this racial group. This chapter describes policy, management, and treatment practices that may enhance access and engagement of African Americans in OUD treatment considering the current opioid epidemic and the state of public treatment systems in the United States. Drawing from a sociocultural framework on disparities in access to care, I present a comprehensive approach based on culturally competent and medication-assisted treatment that may reduce the wait time to enter treatment and increase treatment engagement and recovery rates among African Americans seeking OUD treatment. I focus on the role of public insurance (i.e., Medicaid), the diversification of the workforce, as well as delivery of adequate dosages of maintenance opioid medications (methadone, buprenorphine, and naltrexone) to improve engagement and recovery. Implications for health policy, program design, and service delivery are discussed to abate the effect of the opioid epidemic on African American communities.

Keywords: African Americans, opioid use disorder treatment, Medicaid, cultural competence, treatment effectiveness

1. Introduction

African American communities are disproportionally affected by the opioid epidemic. The CDC estimates that from 2014 to 2016 opioid overdose deaths increased by 45.8% for whites but 83.9% for African Americans [1]. Although white and rural communities have reported alarming overdose rates, African American communities in urban and suburban communities have seen a steady growth of overdoses over a longer period. In particular, the opioid epidemic has disproportionately affected African-American communities, who are most likely than whites to be uninsured or underinsured and unable to enter and stay in opioid use disorder (OUD) treatment.

It is well established that African Americans are more likely than whites to experience difficulty entering and staying in outpatient SUD treatment [2–6]. Researchers have examined wait time to enter treatment and retention in treatment to develop strategies to improve treatment engagement and improve the likelihood of maintaining clients in recovery from opioid use. Wait time to treatment entry is the most commonly cited barrier, and most studies show that African American clients wait more days to enter SUD treatment than non-Hispanic white clients [6–8]. Treatment retention, or time spent in treatment, is a robust predictor of reduced post-treatment substance use [9]. National studies show that treatment programs that provide care to minority populations used fewer approaches to maintain client retention [10–13]. In addition, the importance of insurance coverage to enhance access to OUD treatment for African Americans is noted.

However, since the implementation of the Affordable Care Act, the percentage of clients without insurance in predominately African-American opioid treatment programs (OTPs) dropped from 45% in 2014 to 20% in 2017, which is promising [14, 15]. Delivering culturally responsive care is also critical to engaging African Americans in OUD treatment and reducing the negative effects of the opioid epidemic. In particular, investing in a diverse workforce that is qualified to respond to the technical aspects of medication-assisted treatment and the cultural services needs of African-Americans is critical [16, 17].

The information in this chapter can help policy makers and program managers to make informed decisions about how to allocate scarce resources to help African Americans access effective OUD treatment. Although there are a variety of practices to support treatment access, engagement, and recovery, this chapter focuses on robust approaches to help African Americans considering the current healthcare environment. In this chapter, I describe the evidence supporting Medicaid coverage and delivery of cultural competence in OUD treatment.

2. Cultural competence to enhance access and engagement in OUD treatment for African Americans

Cultural competency is theoretically justified, and mounting evidence supports some of the multiple components or practices to improve engagement and OUD treatment outcomes [18]. However, standardized and empirically validated comprehensive scales through which to measure organizational cultural competence have been lacking [19]. Yet, workforce diversity, which allows matching clients and providers based on language and cultural background and ensuring connections with minority communities have received empirical support [7, 20]. These measures of workforce diversity based on matching have been associated with higher treatment access and retention. A meta-analysis also showed a small, but significant treatment effect of culturally adapted interventions on substance use behaviors among African Americans and Hispanics [21]. This previous research shows promise but requires policy and program investment in tailoring services to the needs of African Americans.

Workforce diversity has become an effective practice to address healthcare disparities in treatment outcomes [22–24]. Following Brach and Fraser, I define workforce diversity as the demographic and cultural representation of health workers and managers that reflect inclusion of backgrounds that are representative of the client population [25]. A diverse workforce is one of the main practices of cultural competence, which is defined as a set of behaviors, attitudes, and policies that enable a system, organization, or individual to function effectively with culturally diverse clients and communities [18]. I draw from the culturally and linguistically appropriate services (CLAS) denomination used by federal health agencies [26–28], which has six main components, Leadership, Quality Improvement and Data Use, Workforce, Patient Safety and Provision of Care, Language Services, and Community Engagement. For a complete list of CLAS practices, please refer to the US Department of Health and Human Services (DHHS), Office of Minority Health. This comprehensive approach describes a healthcare system responsive to the cultural and linguistic service needs of members of racial and ethnic minority individuals.

Workforce diversity as a key practice in CLAS may help OTPs engage African-Americans who are most likely to drop out of treatment. Previous cross-sectional analyses of national representative databases show that SUD treatment programs that cater to minority populations experience decreased retention in treatment or employed methods to maintain retention [9–11, 29, 30]. In contrast, SUD treatment programs with African American supervisors [16] predicted highest degrees of cultural competence. As culturally competent practices can encompass a wide array of organizational arrangements, practices, and services, it is critical for program administrators and counselors to determine which components of CLAS are needed to engage African Americans in OUD treatment.

The importance of diversifying the workforce and delivering CLAS in the SUD treatment system stems from disparate research suggesting that the discordance between the racial background of clients and treatment staff may contribute to health and healthcare disparities [16, 31–34]. Congruence between the cultural and the linguistic backgrounds of staff and clients is thought to elevate the competencies of healthcare providers and improve client treatment adherence via the use of racial/ethnic history and cultural norms, as well as the reliance on client's native language [16, 35–37]. Furthermore, having a diverse workforce may create a conducive climate for implementing CLAS [38, 39] and addressing treatment outcome disparities among minorities [16, 40–42]. The field has seen an increased diversity among SUD clients, but it is not clear how reliably provider/client matching yields positive results [16, 17, 43–45].

Federal, state, and professional organizations have promoted cultural competence to improve SUD treatment engagement (see DHHS Office of Minority Health). Federal regulation, through Medicaid payments of healthcare service has strengthen the focus on delivering services that respond to the cultural and linguistic services needs of clients (DHHS, Medicaid). The National Institute of Medicine, National Institute of Nursing, and the National Association of Social Workers have promoted workforce diversity strategies, as well as developed training standards for cultural competency [46–50]. Regulation at the federal, state, and professional certification levels has incorporated cultural competence in healthcare services [51–54]. More directly to the proposed research, the Substance Abuse and Mental Health Services Administration called providers to rely on CLAS because the majority of SUD counselors are non-Hispanic whites even as almost half who seek treatment are non-white.

Prior research shows that the minority background of managers and counselors is associated with higher rates of treatment access and retention among Latino and African American clients [55–57]. The use of the proposed conceptual framework may expand understanding of drivers of workforce diversity and treatment outcomes. To improve the quality of care provided to African American communities, it is critical to ensure that the different stakeholders understand the service needs of African Americans. This includes engaging policy makers, healthcare administrators, program directors, as well as treatment providers, clients, and people living in the service area who are not clients of the healthcare organization. This comprehensive approach to improve the cultural competency of OUD treatment can have a significant impact on access, retention, and recovery rates of African Americans struggling with OUDs.

3. Medication-assisted treatment and ensuring adequate dosages of opioid maintenance medication

Medication-assisted treatment (MAT) is a pharmacological intervention that relies on specific drugs (e.g., methadone, buprenorphine, or naloxone) to reduce the cravings or block the effects of opioid use. Unfortunately, only one-third of SUD treatment programs offer MAT in the United States, while those opioid treatment programs (OTPs) who provide these medications may not deliver them in adequate dosages compromising the recovery of clients.

Methadone is the most common opioid maintenance medication in the United States. It is used as a replacement for illicit opioid use, such as heroin, in medically supported opioid substitution maintenance programs, referred here as OTPs [58]. Buprenorphine, introduced after methadone, has received significant support to reduce illicit opioid use but has not been widely implemented in OTPs. The effects of buprenorphine may last longer than methadone as it can be taken once every 2 days.

The issue of OTPs providing adequate dosage has been an increasing concern considering the high regulation of medication-assisted programs and the impact on the client population. Emerging research suggests that Methadone doses higher than 60 mg/day are associated with significant declines in heroin consumption [58] and other drug use, as well as with longer retention in treatment and lower rates of relapse [59–63].

However, 41% of patients received lower doses [64] with African Americans more likely to receive doses less than 40 mg/day [17]. This initial findings are concerning as African American communities are disproportionally affected by the opioid epidemic and face significant barriers to access OUD treatment.

Significant evidence shows that buprenorphine at high doses (15 mg) can reduce illicit opioid use effectively [65]. There is limited evidence of African Americans receiving inadequate dosages of buprenorphine, but research has showed that African American communities have less access to buprenorphine treatment compared with White communities.

Adequate dosage of naltrexone is suggested at 50 mg/day [65, 66], but similar to buprenorphine, evidence is limited regarding the adequate dosage of naltrexone in African American communities, while there is some evidence that these communities have less access to naltrexone compared to white communities. Enhancing African American communities' access to MAT and ensuring that maintenance dosages are adequate to maintain recovery should be a primary goal of public health leaders to abate the opioid epidemic.

4. Conceptual framework

The sociocultural framework of substance abuse service disparities [67] suggests that racial disparities in treatment service use originates when healthcare system factors, such as policy, community, and providers differently respond to individuals partly based on their racial/ethnic background. For instance, different stratified conditions emerge when healthcare markets fail in minority communities creating different pathways to access treatment. At the provider level, poor patient-provider communication, lack of trust, and poor workforce availability or competency further differentiates services to minority from services to white clients. As a result of these differences in service provision, racial minorities face greater risk than non-Hispanic whites of dropping out of care and receiving lower quality of care, resulting in worse treatment outcomes [68]. Growing evidence in differences in implementation of health policy in minority communities, provider discrimination, and provider resources offer support for this framework.

I also draw from a diversity and inclusion and funding and regulatory frameworks to describe how racial disparities in OTP may emerge and how to eliminate them. The diversity and inclusion framework proposes that by increasing racial diversity of the OTP workforce, OTPs will be able to be respond to the barriers to access and engagement in treatment [69]. Developing a diverse workforce may enhance OTPs' capacity to deliver CLAS, but OTP's organizational and client factors may determine when OTPs workforce diversity and delivery of culturally responsive care have an impact on process outcomes.

Opioid treatment programs (OTPs) rely heavily on their regulatory and funding environment for financial and nonfinancial (i.e., professional expertise) resources, making them vulnerable to funding and regulatory expectations [7, 70]. OTPs also rely on having a high staff to client ratio to respond to client service needs. The racial/ethnic diversity of the client population is also critical for OTPs to invest in cultural competency and improving process outcomes [16]. These dynamics are consistent with resource-dependence theory [71], which posits that high dependence on necessary resources (Medicaid funding, staffing, and diverse base) determines an organization's practices (e.g., workforce diversity) and selection of core service technologies (e.g., CLAS).

By accepting Medicaid funding, OTPs increase their revenue, but also are pressured to comply with government-endorsed culturally responsive care [72, 73]. Because accepting Medicaid payments may be a proxy for institutional pressures to deliver CLAS and enhance access to healthcare, Medicaid acceptance and the delivery of CLAS may potentially reduce disparities in process outcomes among OTPs primarily serving African Americans and Hispanics. Delivering CLAS may improve OUD treatment programs access, increase retention, and increase percent of clients receiving adequate MAT maintenance dosage when OTPS accept Medicaid payments and when staff/client ratios are high.

Providing African Americans with adequate dosages of methadone, buprenorphine, and or naltrexone is likely to support their commitment to maintenance medication and improve their recovery efforts. A consistent and adequate dosage of these maintenance medications is associated with positive psychosocial, emotional, and labor outcomes. Hence, it is critical to develop the health policies, insurance coverage, service practices, and workforce competencies to deliver culturally responsive and adequate dosing of opioid maintenance medication.

4.1 Organizational factors improving cultural competence and recovery

Prior research on cultural competence in SUD treatment using national data has found that SUD treatment organizations with the highest degree of cultural competence have clinical supervisors and staff who are African American [16]. Studies also show that SUD treatment, when provided using different CLAS, is associated with reduced racial disparities in client access and engagement [7]. For instance, in one of the largest studies on cultural competence, Dr. Guerrero and colleagues included measures from more than 110 treatment organizations and clinical records from 28,000 clients from minority backgrounds. Using these data, they showed that culturally responsive practices are significantly related to client access to treatment services, retention in treatment, and treatment completion [74]. The comprehensive set of organizational practices, (culturally responsive policies and practices, outreach to minority communities, workforce diversity, involvement in minority communities, etc.) make a differences in enhancing treatment access and engagement, as well as ensuring clients meet their treatment plan goals to be successfully discharged.

A critical aspect of OUD treatment is medication dosage. Growing evidence suggests that OTP client characteristics and organizational factors are associated with methadone dose levels [73, 75]. Characteristics of patient mix (percentage of African American patients), employment status (percentage of patients who are currently unemployed), and patient age (percentage of patients aged 40 or above) are associated with dosage levels above 60 mg/day. Program factors associated with methadone dose levels below 60 mgs/day also include program ownership (public, private for profit, and private not-for-profit) accreditation by either the Joint Commission (TJC) or the Commission on Accreditation of Rehabilitation Facilities (CARF), the percentage of staff members who are ex-addicts [75] and African American director, particularly in programs serving populations with higher percentages of African American patients [17, 64, 76]. It is critical to understand the extent to which CLAS may improve OTPs' likelihood of providing adequate MAT dosages in programs serving African American and Latino clients.

Altogether, organizational factors play an important role in the delivery of quality of care for African Americans. When treatment programs provide culturally responsive care, clients engage and respond to treatment. This means that if OTP services are delivered by African American staff with competencies to understand and address the cultural, linguistic, and social service needs of African American clients, these clients are likely to enter, stay, and benefit from OUD treatment.

5. Conclusions

African Americans seeking to enter SUD treatment face significant challenges to engage, stay, and benefit from treatment. Increasing evidence suggests that culturally responsive practices that include workforce diversity as well as policies, practices and services that are responsive to the service needs of African Americans may improve the effectiveness of SUD treatment. African American clients struggling with OUDs may benefit from MAT, in particular three of the most effective medications to address OUD, methadone, buprenorphine, and naltrexone, but ensuring that OTPs deliver MAT, adequate dosages to help African American clients achieve medication maintenance and recovery is critical.

The socio-technical and cultural framework offered in this chapter highlights several factors that may improve treatment of OUD among African Americans. The health policy like Medicaid expansion coverage will ensure effective access to treatment by ensuring ability to pay. This funding also regulates the quality of care, including provision of culturally responsive practices, which include having staff that represent the racial background of clients. The assumption is that the provide-client matching will elevate the cultural understanding of client's OUD issues and address them effectively. The provision of MAT is critical to address OUD, but ensuring adequate dosage of the right type of maintenance medication is necessary. Healthcare system administrators, program managers, and addiction counselors should ensure that African Americans have effective access to the right medication at adequate dosages, and that outcome reporting is available.

5.1 Implications for OUD treatment for African Americans

Opioid use disorder treatment for African Americans may become more effective when investing in program design, a diverse workforce, and MAT. Because research has showed that culturally competent units are typically public, federal-funded organizations and with highly trained staff, in terms of college-educated and professionally certified, it is critical to rely on public funding (Medicaid), professional accreditation standards, and build on staff competencies to deliver OUD treatment that is effective. Culturally competent programs also have a high percent of clients with high severity of illness and social issues [16]. To increase the effectiveness of OUD treatment for an African American population that struggles with other health-related issues, it is critical to integrate MAT and medical services.

Because SUD treatment programs that invest in cultural competence are more likely to invest in ancillary servicessuch as employment counseling, spiritual strength, and physical health, it is also critical for Medicaid reimbursement policies, insurance coverages, program management, and services delivery to respond to the multiple service needs that compromise the recovery of African Americans from opioid use [16, 17].

Policy makers, healthcare administrators, program managers, and counselors need to work conjointly to use their unique knowledge to tailor policies, adjust budgets, design healthcare coverage, and services and prepare the workforce to response to the services needs of African Americans. To reduce the impact of the opioid epidemic on African American communities, public health systems need to improve access to culturally responsive and evidence-based care including effective MAT. Tailoring policies and services to the needs of the racial minority group most represented in OUD treatment has benefit to all members of society.

Acknowledgements

I would like to acknowledge Dr. Thomas D'Aunno for all of his mentorship, assistance, expertise, and collegiality over the many, many years. His support and guidance when I was a student are the primary reasons behind my interest in the topic of African Americans and substance use disorders. I am eternally grateful for the impact that he has had on my professional life.

Conflict of interest

The author declares no conflict of interest.

Thanks

I would like to especially thank Dr. Erick Guerrero for the invitation and opportunity to contribute to this important book.

Acronyms and abbreviations

CARF	Commission on Accreditation of Rehabilitation Facilities
CLAS	culturally and linguistically appropriate services
EBPs	evidence-based practices
NIATx	network for the improvement of addiction treatment
OUD	opioid use disorder
OTP	opioid treatment program
SUD	substance use disorder
TJC	The Joint Commission

Author details

Daniel L. Howard
Texas A&M University, USA

*Address all correspondence to: dannhoward@tamu.edu

References

[1] Bebinger M. 2018. Opioid Overdoses are Rising Faster Among Latinos than Whites or Blacks. Why? Kaiser Health News. May 17, 2018. Available from: https://khn.org/news/opioid-overdoses-are-rising-faster- among-latinos-than-whites-or-blacks-why/

[2] Friedmann PD, Lemon SC, Stein MD, D'Aunno TA. Accessibility of addiction treatment: Results from a national survey of outpatient substance abuse treatment organizations. Health Services Research. 2003;**38**:887-903

[3] Marsh JC, Cao D, Guerrero EG, Shin HC. Need-service matching in substance abuse treatment: Racial/ethnic differences. Evaluation and Program Planning. 2009;**32**:43-51

[4] Tonigan JS. Project match treatment participation and outcome by self-reported ethnicity. Alcoholism: Clinical and Experimental Research. 2003;**27**:1340-1344

[5] Zhang Z, Friedmann PD, Gerstein DR. Does retention matter? Treatment duration and improvement in drug use. Addiction. 2003;**98**:673-684

[6] Andrews CM, Shin HC, Marsh JC, Cao D. Client and program characteristics associated with wait time to substance abuse treatment entry. The American Journal of Drug and Alcohol Abuse. 2013;**39**:61

[7] Guerrero EG. Enhancing access and retention in substance abuse treatment: The role of Medicaid payment acceptance and cultural competence. Drug and Alcohol Dependence. 2013;**132**:555-561. DOI: 10.1016/j.drugalcdep.2013.04.005

[8] Simpson DD, Joe G, Brown B. Treatment retention and follow-up outcomes in the drug abuse treatment outcome study (DATOS). Psychology of Addictive Behaviors. 1997;**11**:294-307

[9] Kleinman PH, Kang SY, Lipton DS, Woody GE, Kemp J, Millman RB. Retention of cocaine abusers in outpatient psychotherapy. American Journal of Alcohol & Drug Abuse. 1992;**18**(1):29-43

[10] Alexander JA, Nahra TA, Lemak CH, Pollack H, Campbell CI. Tailored treatment in the outpatient substance abuse treatment sector: 1995-2005. Journal of Substance Abuse Treatment. Apr 1 2008;**34**(3):282-292

[11] Niv N, Hser YI. Women-only and mixed-gender drug abuse treatment programs: Service needs, utilization and outcomes. Drug and Alcohol Dependence. 2006;**87**(2):194-201. DOI: 10.1016/j.drugalcdep.2006.08.017

[12] Hser YI, Anglin MD, Liu Y. A survival analysis of gender and ethnic differences in responsiveness to methadone maintenance treatment. The International Journal of the Addictions. 1990-1991;**25**:1295-1131

[13] Brown BS, Joe GW, Thompson P. Minority group status and treatment retention. International Journal of the Addictions. 1985;**20**(2):319-335

[14] Grogan CM et al. Survey highlights differences in Medicaid coverage for substance use treatment and opioid use disorder medications. Health Affairs. 2016;**35**(12):2289-2296. http://content.healthaffairs.org/content/35/12/2289.full

[15] Kaiser Foundation. Medicaid's role in addressing the opioid epidemic. The Henry J. Kaiser Family Foundation Headquarters: 2400 Sand Hill Road, Menlo Park, CA 94025 Washington, DC: Kaiser Family Foundation, February 2018. Available from: http://files.kff.org/attachment/infographic-medicaids-role-in-addressing-the-opioid-epidemic

[16] Howard DL. Culturally competent treatment of African American clients among a national sample of outpatient substance abuse treatment units. Journal of Substance Abuse Treatment. 2003a;**24**(2):89-102. DOI: 10.1016/S0740-5472(02)00348-3

[17] Howard DL, Barrett NJ, Holmes DJN. Can cultural competency speak to the race disparities in methadone dosage levels? Review of Black Political Economy. 2010;**37**:7-23

[18] Cross TL, Bazron BJ, Dennis KW, Issacs MR. Towards a Culturally Competent System of Care: Vol. 1. Washington, DC: National Technical Assistance Center for Children's Mental Health; 1989

[19] Harper M, Hernandez M, Nessman T, Mowery D, Worthington J, Issacs M. Organizational Cultural Competence: A Review of Assessment Protocols. Tampa, FL: Research and Training Center for Children's Mental Health, Department of Child and Family Studies, Louis de la Parte Florida Mental Health Institute, College of Behavioral and Community Sciences, University of South Florida; 2009

[20] Guerrero GE, Andrews C. Cultural competence in outpatient substance: Measurement and relationship with wait time and retention. Drug and Alcohol Dependence. 2011;**119**:e13-e22. DOI: 10.1016/j.drugalcdep.2011.05.020

[21] Smith TB, Trimble JE. Foundations of Multicultural Psychology: Research to Inform Effective Practice. Washington, DC: American Psychological Foundation; 2016

[22] Anderson LM, Scrimshaw SC, Fullilove MT, Fielding JE, Normand J, The Task Force on Community Preventive Services. Culturally competent healthcare systems: A systematic review. American Journal of Preventive Medicine. 2003;**24**(3 Suppl):68-79

[23] Hayes-Bautista DE. Research on culturally competent healthcare systems: Less sensitivity, more statistics. American Journal of Preventive Medicine. 2003;**24**(3 Suppl):8-9

[24] Betancourt JR, Green AR, Carrillo JE, Park ER. Cultural competence and health care disparities: Key perspectives and trends. Health Affairs. 2005;**24**(2):499-505

[25] Brach C, Fraser I. Can cultural competency reduce racial and ethnic health disparities? A review and conceptual model. Medical Care Research and Review. 2000;**57**(Suppl 1):181-217

[26] Betancourt JR. Cultural competence—marginal or mainstream movement? The New England Journal of Medicine. 2004;**351**(10):953-955

[27] National Center for Cultural Competence. Definition of Objectives for Organizational Cultural Competence and Service Efficacy. Washington, DC: Center for Child and Human Development, Georgetown University; 2010. Retrieved from: http://nccc.georgetown.edu

[28] U.S. Department of Health and Human Services, Office of Minority Health. National Standards for Culturally and Linguistically Appropriate Services in Health and Health Care: Compendium of State-Sponsored National CLAS Standards Implementation Activities. Washington, DC: U.S. Department of Health and Human Services; 2016

[29] D'Aunno T, Vaughn T. Variation in methadone treatment practices: Results from a national study. Journal of the American Medical Association. 1992;**267**(2):253-258

[30] Wells RB, Lemak CH, D'Aunno T. Organizational survival in the outpatient substance abuse treatment

sector 1988-2000. Medical Care Research and Review. 2005

[31] Bhadury J, Mighty EJ, Damar H. Maximizing workforce diversity in project teams: A network flow approach. Omega. 2000;**28**(2):143-153. DOI: 10.1016/S0305-0483(99)00037-7

[32] Broderick EB. Report to Congress: Addictions Treatment Workforce Development. Washington DC: Substance Abuse and Mental Health Services Administration; 2007

[33] McGuire TG, Miranda J. Racial and ethnic disparities in mental health care: Evidence and policy implications. Health Affairs. 2008;**27**(2):393-403. DOI: 10.1377/hlthaff.27.2.393

[34] Pitts D. Diversity management, job satisfaction, and performance: Evidence from U.S. federal agencies. Public Administration Review. 2009;**69**(2):328-338. DOI: 10.1111/j.1540-6210.2008.01977.x

[35] Grumbach K, Mendoza R. Disparities in human resources: Addressing the lack of diversity in the health professions. Health Affairs. 2008;**27**(2):413-422. DOI: 10.1377/hlthaff.27.2.413

[36] Herring C. Does diversity pay? Race, gender, and the business case for diversity. American Sociological Review. 2009;**74**(2):208-224. DOI: 10.1177/000312240907400203

[37] Lok V, Christian S, Chapman S. Restructuring California's Mental Health Workforce: Interviews with Key Stakeholders. San Francisco. Center for the Health Professions; San Francisco, CA: University of California; 2009

[38] Guerrero EG, Fenwick K, Kong Y. Advancing theory development: Exploring the leadership-climate relationship as a mechanism of the implementation of cultural competence. Implementation Science. 2017;**12**:133

[39] Guerrero GE. Managerial capacity and adoption of culturally competent practices in outpatient substance abuse treatment. Journal of Substance Abuse Treatment. 2010;**39**(4):329-339. DOI: 10.1016/j.jsat.2010.07.004

[40] Prince Inniss JP, Nessman T, Mowery D, Callejas LM, Hernandez M. Serving Everyone at the Table: Strategies for Enhancing the Availability of Culturally Competent Mental Health Service. Tampa, FL: Research and Training Center for Children's Mental Health, Department of Child and Family Studies, Louis de la Parte Florida Mental Health Institute, College of Behavioral and Community Sciences, University of South Florida; 2009

[41] Center for Substance Abuse Treatment. SAMHSA/CSAT Treatment Improvement Protocols. Rockville, MD: Substance Abuse and Mental Health Services Administration; 1993

[42] Center for Substance Abuse Treatment. Addiction Counseling Competencies: The Knowledge, Skills, and Attitudes of Professional Practice. Rockville, MD: Substance Abuse and Mental Health Services Administration; 2006. (TAP Series 21, DHHS Publication No. (SMA) 06-4171)

[43] Quist RM, Law AV. Cultural competency: Agenda for cultural competency using literature and evidence. Research in Social and Administrative Pharmacy. 2006;**2**(3):420-438. DOI: 10.1016/j.sapharm.2006.07.008

[44] Jackson CS, Gracia JN. Addressing health and health-care disparities: The role of a diverse workforce and the social determinants of health. Public Health Reports. 2014;**129**(Suppl 2):57-61

[45] Institute of Medicine. Unequal Treatment: Confronting Racial and Ethnic Disparities in Health Care.

Washington, D.C.: The National Academies Press; 2002

[46] National League for Nursing. A commitment to diversity in nursing and nursing education. Reflections and dialogue. 2009. Available from: http://www.nln.org/about/position-statements/nln-reflections-dialogue/read/dialoguereflection/2009/01/02/reflection-dialogue-3-

[47] National League for Nursing. Percentage of minority students enrolled in basic RN programs: 1995, 2005, 2009 to 2012, and 2014. NLN biennial survey of schools; 2014

[48] Olinger BH. Increasing nursing workforce diversity: Strategies for success. Nurse Educator. 2011;**36**(2):54-55. DOI: 10.1097/NNE.0b013e31820b4fab

[49] U.S Department of Health and Human Services. Health Resources and Services Administration. Pipeline programs to improve racial and ethnic diversity in the health professions. 2009. Retrieved from http://bhpr.hrsa.gov/healthworkforce/reports/pipelineprogdiversity.pdf

[50] Department of Health and Human Services. Strategic Plan. 2015. Available from: https://www.hhs.gov/sites/default/files/secretary/about/priorities/strategicplan2010-2015.pdf

[51] National Association of Social Workers. Cultural Competence Standards in Social Work. Available from: https://www.socialworkers.org/LinkClick.aspx?fileticket=PonPTDEBrn4%3D&portalid=0 [Accessed: Feb 5, 2019]

[52] New Jersey Standards of Practice. Cultural Competence. Available from: https://www.njleg.state.nj.us/2004/Bills/PL05/53_.HTM [Accessed: Feb 5, 2019]

[53] Substance Abuse and Mental Health Service Administration. Effective Practices with Racial/Ethnic Minorities. Available from: https://store.samhsa.gov/shin/content/SMA14-4849/SMA14-4849.pdf [Accessed: Feb 5, 2019]

[54] Joint Commission. 2012. Office of Minority Health National Culturally and Linguistically Appropriate Services (CLAS) Standards Crosswalked to Joint Commission 2007 Standards for Hospitals, Ambulatory, Behavioral Health, Long Term Care, and Home Care [Online information; retrieved December 31, 2007]. Available from: www.jointcommission.org/NR/rdonlyres/5EABBEC8-F5E2-4810-A16F-E2F148AB5170/0/hlc_omh_xwalk.pdf

[55] Guerrero GE, Andrews C. Cultural competence in outpatient substance abuse treatment: Measurement and relationship with wait time and retention. Drug and Alcohol Dependence. 2011;**119**:e13-e22. DOI: 10.1016/j.drugalcdep.2011.05.020

[56] Guerrero EG, Khachikian T, Kim T, Kong Y, Vega WA. Spanish language proficiency among providers and Latino clients' engagement in substance abuse treatment. Addictive Behaviors. 2013;**38**(12):2893-2897

[57] Guerrero EG, Garner B, Cook B, Kong Y. Does the implementation of evidence based and culturally competent practices reduce disparities in addiction treatment outcomes? Addictive Behaviors. 2017;**73**:119-123

[58] Baumeister M, Vogel M, Dürsteler-MacFarland KM, Gerhard U, Strasser J, Walter M, et al. Association between methadone dose and concomitant cocaine use in methadone maintenance treatment: a register-based study. Substance Abuse Treatment, Prevention, and Policy. 2014;**9**:46. DOI: 10.1186/1747-597X-9-46

[59] Brady TM, Salvucci S, Sverdlov LS, Male A, Kyeyune H, Sikali E, et al. Methadone dosage and retention:

An examination of the 60 mg/day threshold. Journal of Addictive Diseases. 2005;**24**(3):23-47

[60] Donny EC, Brasser SM, Bigelow GE, Stitzer ML, Walsh SL. Methadone doses of 100 mg or greater are more effective than lower doses at suppressing heroin self-administration in opioid-dependent volunteers. Addiction. 2005;**100**(10):1496-1509

[61] Fareed A, Casarella J, Roberts M, Sleboda M, Amar R, Vayalapalli S, et al. High dose versus moderate dose methadone maintenance: Is there a better outcome? Journal of Addictive Diseases. 2009;**28**(4):399-405

[62] Fareed A, Casarella J, Amar R, Vayalapalli S, Drexler K. Methadone maintenance dosing guideline for opioid dependence, a literature review. Journal of Addictive Diseases. 2010;***29***(1):1-14

[63] Yan-ping B, Liu Z-M, Epstein DH, Cun D, Jie S, Lin L. A meta-analysis of retention in methadone maintenance by dose and dosing strategy. American Journal of Drug & Alcohol Abuse. 2009;**35**(1):28-33

[64] D'Aunno T, Park SE, Pollack HA. Evidence-based treatment for opioid use disorders: A national study of methadone dose levels, 2011-2017. Journal of Substance Abuse Treatment. Jan 1 2019;**96**:18-22

[65] Dowell D, Haegerich TM, Chou R. CDC guideline for prescribing opioids for chronic pain—United States, 2016. JAMA. 2016;**315**(15):1624-1645

[66] Kampman K, Jarvis M. American Society of Addiction Medicine (ASAM) national practice guideline for the use of medications in the treatment of addiction involving opioid use. Journal of Addiction Medicine. 2015;**9**(5):358

[67] Alegría M, Pescosolido BA, Canino G. A socio-cultural framework for mental health and substance abuse service disparities. In: Sadock BJ, Sadock VA, Ruiz P, editors. *Kaplan & Sadock's Comprehensive Textbook of Psychiatry*. 9th ed. Philadelphia, PA: Lippincott Williams & Wilkins; 2009. pp. 4370-4379

[68] McCaul ME, Svikis DS, Moore RD. Predictors of outpatient treatment retention: Patient versus substance use characteristics. Drug and Alcohol Dependence. 2001;***62***(1):9-17

[69] Guerrero GE. Workforce diversity in outpatient substance abuse treatment: The role of leaders' characteristics. Journal of Substance Abuse Treatment. 2013;**44**(2):208-215. DOI: 10.1016/j.jsat.2012.05.004

[70] D'Aunno T. The role of organization and management in substance abuse treatment: Review and roadmap. Journal of Substance Abuse Treatment. 2006;**31**(3):221-233

[71] Pfeffer J, Salancik GR. *The External Control of Organizations*. New York, NY: Harper & Row; 1978

[72] Schmidt LA, Ye Y, Greenfield TK, Bond J. Ethnic disparities in clinical severity and services for alcohol problems: Results from the National Alcohol Survey. Alcoholism: Clinical and Experimental Research. 2007;**31**:48-56

[73] D'Aunno T, Pollack H. Changes in methadone treatment practices: Results from a national study, 1988-2000. Journal of the American Medical Association. 2002;**288**(7):850-857

[74] Guerrero EG, Aarons GA, Grella CE, Garner BR, Cook B, Vega WA. Program capacity to eliminate outcome disparities in addiction health services. Administration and Policy in Mental Health and Mental Health Services Research. 2016;**43**(1):23-35

[75] D'Aunno T, Pollack HA, Frimpong JA, Wuchiett D. Evidence-based treatment for opioid disorders: A 23-year national study of methadone dose levels. Journal of Substance Abuse Treatment. 2014;**47**(4):245-250. DOI: 10.1016/j.jsat.2014.06.001

[76] Frimpong JA, Shiu-Yee K, D'Aunno T. The role of program directors in treatment practices: The case of methadone dose patterns in U.S. outpatient opioid agonist treatment programs. Health Services Research. 2017;**52**(5):1881-1907. DOI: 10.1111/1475-6773.12558

Section 4

Approaches to Improve System Effectiveness

Chapter 5

Management Practices to Enhance the Effectiveness of Substance Use Disorder Treatment

Jemima A. Frimpong and Erick G. Guerrero

Abstract

Managers of substance use disorder (SUD) treatment organizations face significant challenges to improve treatment effectiveness. The field has paid significant attention to the delivery of pharmacological and psychosocial treatment interventions, and the effectiveness of these interventions, with little consideration for the role of management practices that enhance the delivery of such evidence-based practices (EBPs). This chapter describes evidence-based management practices (EBMPs) that may support the effective and consistent delivery of EBPs in SUD treatment. Drawing from a socio-technical and cultural framework, we propose a management approach that relies on policies, human resources, and culturally responsive practices to directly and or indirectly facilitate the delivery of EBPs. In particular, this chapter describes EBMPs that could be widely implemented to respond to the cultural, linguistic, and service needs of racial and ethnic minority groups. We discuss implications for funding and support of management training to improve standards of care and include a case example to promote reflection.

Keywords: evidence-based management practices, effectiveness, workforce diversity, substance use disorder treatment

1. Introduction

Evidence-based management practices (EBMPs) are grounded on evidence with significant empirical support to facilitate organizational change and performance improvement [1, 2]. As such, EBMP refers to meso and macro practices that may enhance the effectiveness of micro practices (e.g., EBPs or interventions at the practitioner-client level). Emerging evidence suggest that EBMPs play an important role in the effectiveness of behavioral health services by supporting the process of service delivery [3–6]. EBMPs are therefore increasingly important to respond to the high demand for public accountability, organizational performance and implementation fidelity in health and human services [7].

The substance use disorder (SUD) treatment field has focused on clinical interventions that show effectiveness in reducing substance use. In particular, there has been significant development of EBPs in the use of medication and psychosocial interventions to reduce substance use or support abstinence. Yet, there is limited application of evidence-based management practices (EBMPs) that support the delivery and integration of EBPs into routine practice. Once an intervention is considered effective, it is critical to understand the contextual factors that play a role in supporting effectiveness in the delivery and continued use of the intervention.

Management in SUD treatment organizations are a complex and multifaceted practice that seeks to improve the structure, technology and human resource capacity to enhance service delivery and achieve positive treatment outcomes [8]. Managers consequently play a critical role to develop, implement, and sustain EBPs [9, 10]. Although managers tend to rely on personal experience to inform practices used in their organizations, it is critical to develop management capacity to rely on EBMP to enhance the impact of EBPs in SUD treatment [5, 11].

Managers in SUD treatment organizations face significant challenges to increase access to care and ensure high rates of recovery from SUD. Among the most documented challenges to enhance access to effective care include preparing the workforce to deliver culturally responsive and evidence-based treatment [12, 13], develop a sustainable funding approach and relying on technology to track staff performance and client progress. To do so, managers need to rely on best practices in human resources, finance and staff and client progress measurement [12, 14–16]. The field of management in SUD treatment could benefit from more than 100 years of management research. Drawing from this discipline, there are at least three EBMPs that could improve the effective implementation of EBPs in SUD treatment. The management practices with significant evidentiary bases include: (1) goal setting, (2) feedback and redesign models, and (3) total quality management. Our emphasis on these practices, among the range of evidence-based management practices, is grounded on the context of social service organizations. Specifically, these practices are relevant to the organizational challenges most implicated in the effective delivery of substance use disorder treatment, and challenges where they are mostly to have impact. We select these practices in line with the unique challenges faced by managers in substance use disorder treatment programs (e.g., organizational capacity, staffing) [17]. These management practices also consider various levels of challenges, i.e., development/pre-implementation: establishing alignment between expected outcomes and goals by putting in place systems that support the outcome; testing/implementation: a double-loop approach to learning and adapting to change; and continuous/post- implementation: engaging staff at all levels of program to ensure maintenance of effectiveness and quality.

2. Evidence-based management practices

Goal-setting is defined as a motivational technique that is used to set specific goals that will enhance performance, with more-difficult goals resulting in higher performance [18]. Goals help motivate individuals to accomplish challenging objectives by establishing specific and measurable targets. Research on goal-setting practice has further suggested that when team members work together towards a common goal, it helps ensure that the goal will be achieved [18]. Goal-setting as a practice has its limitations because it does not take into consideration the factor of time [19]. For instance, in an organization, accomplishing a given goal, and specifically by a certain specified time, may not be aligned with supervisors' overall assessment of when the set goal is to be realized, or the organizations expectations for the goal. This misalignment has implications for how tasks and resources are prioritized and managed over time. As a result, varying understanding and expectation of time horizons may create direct conflict between employers and employees within the organization, and thus lead to weakness in overall performance. Aligning priorities and setting realistic timelines are among the many issues that managers need to address to benefit from the goal-setting practice.

Goal setting is however an EBMP that could be implemented in SUD Treatment organizations. Although this practice requires training and persistence in the supervisor-counselor relationship, it does not require an elaborate plan, costly resources, or a complex structure. It requires managers' careful assessment of staff members' strengths and limitations, as well as the facilitators and barriers to ensure a successful service outcome. The practice is also alike the treatment planning process that counselors review with clients to support their positive treatment outcomes, such as sobriety. Considering its low-cost, simplicity and ease of implementation, this practice is highly recommended for SUD treatment settings.

Feedback and redesign model is a more comprehensive EBMP, which considers four steps: context, behavior, impact, and future steps. Context describes the situation in which the individual is allotted time to provide feedback [20]. In the next phase, the individual describes their behavior, given the context, as clearly as possible, to draw conclusions. This has an impact of the situation, and the feedback may be positive or negative. The nature of the impact then leads to discussions of specific behaviors to determine if a redesign or change should be implemented. The interconnectedness of the analysis between feedback and redesign can then be used by managers to help individuals plan, evaluate, and overcome challenges [21].

The feedback and redesign model offers managers of SUD treatment services the opportunity to comprehensively assess micro and meso level factors that play a role in accomplishing the desired goal. Managers may use this model in clinical supervision, where counselor-client context, and counselor's intervention and desired outcome are constantly the focus. This model has informed well-known interventions such as the Plan-Do-Study-Act (PDSA) cycle. The PDSA approach relies on a scientific method applied to action-oriented learning. The goal is that to test isolated changes, organizations need to plan the change, try it, observe the results, and act on what is learned. Researchers have pilot tested this intervention in several studies to enhance treatment access and retention. The Network for the Improvement of Addiction Treatment (NIATx) model [22] uses a Plan-Do-Study-Act (PDSA) cycle. This cycle is designed to identify issues and create solutions (Plan), implement new processes (Do), evaluate outcomes (Study), and establish change practices (Act) [23, 24]. In the public health system in Los Angeles County, researchers have tested the PDSA approach to improve treatment retention with positive results [25].

The Plan-Do-Study-Act can be resource intensive, particularly for small treatment organizations that lack the guidance, personnel and time to implement such rigorous cycles. But, there is increasing support from government and foundations to help small treatment organization form coalitions to support PDSAs in their communities. As such, the PDSA can be considered a EBMP that could improve the effectiveness of SUD treatment.

Total quality management (TQM) or continuing quality management (CQM) model is another model with supportive evidence to improve service effectiveness. Coined by William Edwards Deming [26], total quality management (TQM) is defined as a system of management that views every staff member of an organization as responsible for maintaining the highest standards of work within every aspect of the organization's operation. TQM is used in organizations to help improve procedures in all areas of functionality [27]. TQM has become a popular management approach because it strives to improve product quality and interactions with customers and suppliers, which are linked to organizational design and change. Subsequently, the quality of a business has become an important aspect of an organization's success. Although TQM is prevalent within organizations, it requires extensive training. This approach has been mainly used and tested in manufacturing, with little exposure to health and human services. Studies focusing on health care have sought to integrate TQM into a continuing quality management framework applied to healthcare. Existing evidence suggests significant benefits of implementing this framework in healthcare services [28].

Although the TQM, or CQM perspective can be resource intensive, it may allow SUD treatment systems to examine more broadly every aspect of the process of care. This approach can be used by state or county level administrator of healthcare services to guide quality improvement efforts. For instance, TQM can be applied to each step in the process of care, which may be divided by phases—e.g., outreach, intake, assessment, treatment planning, discharge, continuing of care. The culmination of efforts within each phase would then factor into improved service delivery and effectiveness.

3. Evidence-based management in SUD treatment organizations

The SUD treatment field has gradually built a series of EBMPs informed by managers' experience, and the continuous need to respond to a complex regulatory and funding environment. For instance, under health care reform, SUD treatment organizations are expected to become more systematic in service delivery and accountable to service outcomes, requiring the use of EBMPs to support the implementation, delivery, and effectiveness of EBPs.

The concept of evidence-based health care has led to a significant shift in the way health care professionals use evidence from scientific research and practice. Managers often encourage drug treatment counselors to adopt an EBP approach to practice, yet managers in SUD treatment often lack formal education in management, or the managerial capacity to rely on EBMPs to support delivery of EBPs [11]. The increased interest in developing EBP in the management of health care organizations is mainly due to wide variation in the implementation and effect of clinical EBPs [29].

The selection, implementation, sustainment, and influence of effective EBPs depend on how health care services are financed, regulated and delivered [11]. Leaders of health and social services system have begun to call for translation of findings from behavioral economics, cognitive and social psychology, management science, and social work, among other disciplines, to inform EBMPs [30]. Communities of scientist, academicians, and practitioners have also been encouraged to work together to translate current management practices with significant evidence, as well as to invest in the development of practical responses to current management challenges [30]. As such, practitioners will not need to rely on personal experience and local knowledge to address challenges that stem from principles addressed in research and science. We extend the socio-technical framework [12] of SUD treatment systems and include a cultural aspect to respond to the cultural and linguistic service needs of racial/ethnic minority clients. This social-technical framework posits that community and organizational factors enhance access to treatment services and the use of EBPs [18]. We categorized EBMPs relevant to SUD treatment organizations into four main areas: *Policy, Social, Technical and Cultural Practices.* These practices operate at different levels to impact organizational and treatment level outcomes.

4. Management practices that rely on policy factors

The policy context of SUD treatment is critical to determine whether a policy initiative can be evidence-based to enhance access to care [11]. The Affordable Care Act (ACA) legislation abolished categorical restrictions on eligibility for Medicaid that have traditionally limited enrollment to children, parents, and individuals with qualifying disabilities. By removing insurance restrictions and thus, reducing financial barriers, these ACA changes have the potential to improve access to substance abuse treatment [31, 32]. Hispanics are at the highest risk of being uninsured, with non-elderly adult Hispanics nearly two and half times as likely to be uninsured than non-elderly adult Whites (22 vs. 9%). Since the implementation of the ACA, the percentage of clients without insurance in predominately African-American OTPs dropped from 45% in 2014 to 20% in 2017; similarly, this percentage dropped from 49% in 2014 to 27% in 2017 in predominately Hispanic programs. Because Medicaid expansion was deemed optional after the ruling in National Federal of Independent Business *v. Sebelius*, gains in insurance access and, in turn, treatment access, has been shown only in states that chose to open program eligibility to all low-income adults [33].

Management practices that rely on policy changes or practices, such as the ACA, can significantly improve access to care for under-represented population groups, including Hispanics and African-Americans, who remain more likely to be uninsured than Whites. Medicaid expansion and program acceptance of Medicaid reduces barriers to access treatment for racial and ethnic minority groups [34]. This is because SUD treatment programs are motivated to admit individuals to treatment to the extent that they have insurance coverage. We thus highlight Medicaid expansion as evidence-based policy practice.

5. Management practices that rely on social factors

5.1 Staff to client ratios

Prior work shows that staff to client ratio is an important predictor of the use of evidence-based practices in the nation's SUD treatment programs [35]. As this ratio increases, clients are more likely to receive medical and social services [12]. The likely mechanism in this relationship is staff time devoted to clients. That is, when caseloads increase, staff member simply does not have the time to respond adequately to clients' service needs, including, for example, making referral arrangements to link clients to needed services that are often located off-site [36]. Effective management of staff to client ratios can be considered an EBMPs that may support quality of care, particularly for vulnerable clients that need integrated care services.

6. Management practices that rely on technical factors

Resources available to SUD treatment programs are likely to play an important role in their behavior. Workforce, (staff-client ratios) technology (use of electronic health records), and quality improvement initiatives (accreditation) as resources, are therefore catalysts for the use of EBPs.

6.1 Financing models

Due to fewer financial resources, programs that serve higher percentages of minority clients are less likely to have or use electronic health records (EHRs). Prior work shows that EHRs play an important role in managing and coordinating client care, especially linking clients in substance abuse treatment to mainstream health care providers [37, 38]. For example, programs with high percentages of minority clients rely heavily on public funds (Medicaid reimbursement and state block grants) which provide lower levels of financial support to cover expenses for their operations—including payroll for staff salaries; funds to purchase and maintain information technology systems for electronic health records; and funds for staff training and quality improvement programs. In comparison, programs that serve higher percentages of white clients might have, on average, more funding from private insurance, client self-pay, and donations. These funding sources might enable support for the integration of more EBPs like medical and mental health services, as well as the linkage with social services and the provision of aftercare services. Having EHRs may also be considered a management practices to enhance quality of care [35]. Hence, diversifying funding streams and increasing revenue from private insurance, self-pay and donations can be considered a management practice that can directly enhance the delivery of EBPs.

6.2 Professional accreditation

Prior research shows that SUD treatment programs that hold accreditation from the Joint Commission (TJC) are more likely to provide higher quality of care [12, 39]. Attaining accreditation from TJC is resource-intensive but programs with TJC are held accountable to provide EBPs. Program efforts to respond to accreditation standards seem to play a significant role in supporting the effectiveness of EBPs. Through the gaining and sustaining professional accreditation, managers may be able to invest in processes that support effectiveness. Having the necessary technical resources to improve the quality of care may contribute to the effectiveness of SUD treatment.

7. Management practices that rely on cultural factors

7.1 Workforce diversity

Growing evidence suggests that clients from racial and ethnic minority backgrounds respond more favorably to treatment staff who share their cultural and linguistic background [40–47]. Although cultural humility and respect for clients' cultural background is critical for services, most of the literature has examined provider-client matching as an initial condition to improve treatment engagement. Workforce diversity is one of the most concrete practices that represent organizational cultural competence. Workforce diversity generally indicates whether treatment staff, including directors, supervisors and counselors are reflective and representative of their client population, i.e., members of a minority group (e.g., African American or Hispanic) [42, 48]. Prior research on workforce diversity shows that SUD treatment programs identified as culturally competent are much more likely than other programs to have clinical supervisors and staff who are African American [49]. Supervisors and directors of culturally competent programs may have important attributes that may help engage minority clients. Research shows that those managers working in programs with high cultural competence also report graduate education and significant work experience. Hence, workforce diversity may also bring highly skilled, educated, trained, and experienced managers and staff who can competently respond to the cultural service needs of clients.

The extant literature on SUD treatment systems across the country show that when minority counselors provide services, minority clients enter treatment faster than when serviced by White counselors [47, 49–52]. For instance, culturally responsive policies, management and service practices are associated with greater retention in treatment; and treatment completion [42, 53]. The organizational context underlying practices that are responsive to the cultural diversity of the population served, especially in social service organizations, cannot be understated. Specifically, the multidimensional aspect of factors that facilitate effective response to diverse population, at the program level, include: a multicultural service delivery philosophy (e.g., partnerships with local agencies, reducing duplication of services that are costly); responsive organizational processes (e.g., collaboration with agencies with similar goals, considering limited resources); responsive organizational procedures (e.g., managerial support for policies that illustrate mission statement and service standards); continuous organizational renewal (e.g., ongoing needs assessments); and effective agency-community relations (e.g., the establishment of relationships that are not grounded on power dynamics) [54]. Thus, culturally responsive practices can be considered EBMPs when used in management to enhance client outcomes. These results have informed policy interventions to invest in translation of materials, diversification of the workforce and counselors' Spanish language proficiency [53]. Despite this evidence, workforce diversity national initiatives require more financial, legislative and social support to improve the treatment conditions for members of racial and ethnic minority groups entering the SUD treatment system.

8. Implications for managers in SUD treatment organizations

EBMPs described in this chapter are not exhaustive of all practices available, nor are they fully described for training purposes. They are however some of the most significant practices based on the current context of healthcare reform in the United States and the increasing participation of racial and ethnic minority clients entering the SUD treatment system. Our goals for this chapter was to bring awareness to policy makers, health care administrators, program managers and other stakeholders of a series of evidence-based practices that can improve the effectiveness of SUD treatment.

Because most managers of SUD treatment are generally promoted from direct service provider (i.e., counselor) to middle manager (clinical supervisor) and sometimes to program director, it is critical to train them on the job. These man agers also have limited formal education in the latest management theories and practices that makes them effective as managers of healthcare services. Federal, State and Foundations should require and financially support comprehensive management training for all SUD treatment programs, nationwide [55]. Such trainings should focus on a package of training that focus on, but not limited to the transition to management and leadership, role identity, and the necessary knowledge and skills, in order to solidly prepare former clinicians on astute implementers of EBMPs. The extent, as well as implementation of a comprehensive training agenda will in turn make progress on the ongoing efforts to professionalize the field. Treatment programs would accordingly function with evidence-based practices at the core of their operations. This will be reinforced by the knowledge and experiences of providers, which would benefit clients who demand high quality, efficient, effective, and cost-effectiveness care to address their substance use disorder.

9. Case example

Lorena Perez was one of the most popular, active and friendly managers in her human service organization. She managed their substance use disorder treatment division, which included several inpatient and outpatient treatment programs in the suburbs of a large city on the East Coast. Ms. Perez did not receive any formal training in management. In fact, she started as a client in one of the inpatient programs 30 years ago. After completing the program and maintaining her sobriety from alcohol, Ms. Perez first volunteered as a sponsor to many Latino women in recovery. After a few years, she completed her Bachelors' degree in Psychology and addictions and became certified as a substance abuse counselor. She was given a full-time job in the same program that helped her recover. During her 10 years as a counselor, she became one of the most effective counselors engaging hundreds of women in the process of recovery. Although she relied heavily on her recovery experience and 12 step approach, she incorporated this approach with the latest evidence-based interventions to her individual and group counseling. Ms. Perez was always eager to attend trainings to improve her skills and competencies in all areas of the treatment process. After a few years, her personal commitment to effectiveness, was noticed by the organization's leaders, and Ms. Perez was promoted to clinical supervisor.

With no formal management experience, Ms. Perez struggled to provide counselors with effective support. She treated counselors under her direction as clients, spending a great deal of time processing their emotions and supporting their decision making. Even though staff felt emotionally supported, which had a positive effect on their view of the relationship with Ms. Perez, they did not have a sense of what they were working towards, both at a personal and program levels. They knew that with more guidance, they could better serve their clients, and further improve the functioning of the organization. With these looming gaps, the treatment staff became increasingly frustrated with her supervisory and approach to management. These dynamics were compounded by resource constraints that Ms. Perez had to operate within. She finds herself managing a program and team, but did not have the necessary resources to meaningfully engage her staff. This meant that she often had to reschedule or cancel one-on-one review meetings and program-wide meetings. These missed opportunities for engagement meant that staff did not get needed critical feedback on their performance or ways in which they may improve their performance. It also meant that she did not get to learn about and address challenges faced by staff in the care delivery process. Within the broader organizational context, Mrs. Perez also had fewer touch-points with clients. These interactions, she has also found to be invaluable to her experience and knowledge as a practitioner and manager. Because of her lessened presence, with respect to client-facing interactions, she began to lose track of the changing patient demographic and did not always consider alignment between the population that the program is serving, and the staff. In the end, although the staff felt emotionally supported, they requested practical guidance on how to become more effective in the process of care (e.g., screening, intake, assessment, counseling, discharge) and improve performance. Ms. Perez also knew that changes were necessary, for her to be successful in her role as a manager, and improve performance.

Ms. Perez requested help from upper management. She wanted to either go back to counseling clients, which she knew well and was clearly effective, or to receive training to become an effective manager for her team.

Discussion questions:

1. Why was Ms. Perez not successful in helping her team become more effective?

2. What evidence-based practice are available to Ms. Perez, as a manager to help her team achieve their performance goals?

3. What can Ms. Perez do to help her team follow an evidence-based process that leads to better treatment results, i.e., how the process be operationalized to comprehensively improve performance?

4. What may be other approaches to improve the diversity of the program and improve cultural competency?

10. Conclusion

The field of SUD treatment has focused on delivery of evidence-based pharmaceutical and psychosocial interventions with little attention to the management practices that support the implementation of such EBPs. The field can benefit from evidence-based management practices (EBMP) to increase the effectiveness of EBPs. SUD treatment organizations could benefit from EBMP with different degrees of investment. For instance, goal setting is an easier practice to implement and generally with low cost, while the feedback and redesign model requires more resources and organization but may improve system functioning. The total quality management, also referred as continuing quality management model is the most resource-intense EBMPs presented here, but one that can result in significant and sustained system change. Managers of SUD treatment programs with the appropriate training on these models, can apply these concepts to their context and improve treatment effectiveness.

Instead of solely relying on managers' experience and common sense, the field seeks to improve managers' decision making by relying on many of the practices described in this chapter. Although this was not intended as an exhaustive list of EBMPs, we selected practices that seem to benefit the SUD treatment field, because they are either analogous to existing treatment practices (e.g. goal setting in treatment planning or in development) or easily implementable.

Other EBMPs that have developed as a response to the funding and regulatory context of SUD treatment are policy initiatives like accepting Medicaid payments and obtaining premier professional certifications. Although most SUD treatment programs in the United States are small, with 3 to 5 counselors and less than 1 million dollars in revenue yearly, these programs are now considering forming coalitions to guide, support and maintain premier certification standards and implement system wide continuing quality management.

Standalone EBMPs are also available for managers of SUD treatment services. Implementing an Electronic Health Record system is critical to track progress and show improvement in quality of care and effectiveness. Managers could consider again the benefit of having their own EHR system, or collaborating with larger treatment organizations to benefit from their systems. Similarly, applying innovative human resources practices, managers can overcome staff recruitment, retention and promotion with the right guidance and resources. Finally, developing a culturally responsive treatment program requires astute management practices to diversify, train and support their staff on culturally responsive care. Although these practices are often singularly implemented, managers can rely on the EBMPs framework to support their efforts to improve treatment effectiveness.

Acknowledgements

We would like to acknowledge the support from the Integrated Substance Abuse Treatment to Eliminate Disparities research team.

Conflict of interest

The author declares no conflict of interest.

Abbreviations

EBMPs	evidence-based management practices
EBPs	evidence-based practices
NIATx	Network for the Improvement of Addiction Treatment
OUD	opioid use disorder
OTP	opioid treatment program
SUD	substance use disorder
TJC	the Joint Commission

Author details

Jemima A. Frimpong[1*] and Erick G. Guerrero[2]

1 Carey Business School, Johns Hopkins University, Baltimore, MD, United States

2 I-Lead Institute, Research to End Healthcare Disparities Corp, Santa Monica, CA, United States

*Address all correspondence to: jafrimpong@jhu.edu

References

[1] Mullen PM. Using performance indicators to improve performance. Health Services Management Research. 2004;**17**:217-228

[2] Ohmer ML. Assessing and developing the evidence base of macro practice interventions with a community and neighborhood focus. Journal of Evidence-Based Social Work. 2008;**5**:519-547. DOI: 10.1080/15433710802084284

[3] Aarons GA, Hurlburt M, Horwitz SM. Advancing a conceptual model of evidence-based practice implementation in public service sectors. Administration and Policy in Mental Health. 2011;**38**:4-23

[4] Gray RM. Addictions and the self: A self-enhancement model for drug treatment in the criminal justice system. Journal of Social Work Practice in the Addictions. 2001;**1**:75-91. DOI: 10.1300/J160v01n02_07

[5] Guerrero EG. Managerial capacity and adoption of culturally competent practices in outpatient substance abuse treatment. Journal of Substance Abuse Treatment. 2010;**39**:329-339. DOI: 10.1016/j.jsat.2010.07.004

[6] Norcross J, Levant R, Beutler L. Evidence-Based Practices in Mental Health: Debate and Dialogue on the Fundamental Questions. Washington, DC: American Psychological Association Press; 2005

[7] Briggs HE, McBeath B. Evidence-based management: Origins, challenges, and implications for social service administration. Administration in Social Work. 2009;**33**:242-261. DOI: 10.1080/03643100902987556

[8] Patti RJ. The Handbook of Human Services Management. 2nd ed. Thousand Oaks, CA: Sage; 2009

[9] Sackett DL, Straus SE, Richardson WS, Rosenberg W, Haynes RB. Evidence- Based Medicine: How to Practice and Teach EBM. 2nd ed. London, England: Churchill Livingstone; 2000

[10] Abrahamson E. Management fashion. Academy of Management Review. 1996;**21**:254-285. DOI: 10.5465/AMR.1996.9602161572

[11] Frimpong JA, Shiu-Yee K, D'Aunno T. The role of program directors in treatment practices: The case of methadone dose patterns in U.S. outpatient opioid agonist treatment programs. Health Services Research. 2016;**52**(5):1881-1907. DOI: 10.1111/1475-6773.12558

[12] D'Aunno T. The role of organization and management in substance abuse treatment: Review and roadmap. Journal of Substance Abuse Treatment. 2006;**31**:221-233

[13] Guerrero GE. Managerial challenges and strategies to implementing organizational change in substance abuse treatment for Latinos. Administration in Social Work. 2013;**37**:286-296. DOI: 10.1080/03643107.2012.686009

[14] McLellan AT, Carise D, Kleber HD. Can the national addiction treatment infrastructure support the public's demand for quality care? Journal of Substance Abuse Treatment. 2003;**25**(2):117-121. DOI: 10.1016/S0740-5472(03)00156-9

[15] Center for Substance Abuse Treatment (CSAT). Clinical supervision and professional development of the substance abuse counselor. Treatment Improvement Protocol (TIP) Series 52, DHHS Publication No. (SMA) 09-4377. Rockville, MD: Substance Abuse and Mental Health Administration; 2009a

[16] Center for Substance Abuse Treatment (CSAT). Implementing change in substance abuse treatment programs. Treatment Improvement Protocol (TIP) Series 31, DHHS Publication No. (SMA) 09-4377. Rockville, MD: Substance Abuse and Mental Health Administration; 2009b

[17] Austin MJ, Regan K, Samples M, Schwartz S, Carnochan S. Building managerial and organizational capacity in nonprofit human service organizations through a leadership development program. Administration in Social Work. 2011;**35**(3):258-281

[18] Rousseau DM. 2005 presidential address: Is there such a thing as evidence-based management? Academy of Management Review. 2006;**31**:256-269

[19] Menefee ML, Vandeveer RC. Human Behavior in Organizations. 2nd ed. Upper Saddle River, NJ: Prentice Hall; 2009

[20] Kovner AR, Elton JJ, Billings JD. Evidence-based management. Frontiers of Health Services Management. 2005;**16**:3-24

[21] Locke EA, Latham GP. Goal Setting: A Motivational Technique that Works. Englewood Cliffs, NJ: Prentice-Hall; 1984

[22] McCarty D, Gustafon DH, Wisdom JP, Ford J, Choi D, Molfenter T, et al. The network for the improvement of addiction treatment (NIATx): Enhancing access and retention. Drug and Alcohol Dependence. 2007;**88**:138-145

[23] Gitlow H, Gitlow S, Oppenheim A, Oppenheim R. Tools and Methods for the Improvement of Quality. Homewood, IL: Irwin; 1989

[24] Shewart WA. Statistical Method from the Viewpoint of Quality Control. Lancaster, PA: Lancaster Press; 1939

[25] Rutkowshi BA, Gallon S, Rawson RA, Freese TE, Bruehl A, Crevecoeur MacPhail D, et al. Improving client engagement and retention in treatment: The Los Angeles County experience. Journal of Substance Abuse Treatment. 2010;**39**:78-86

[26] Locke EA, Latham GP. What should we do about motivation theory? Six recommendations for the twenty-first century. Academy of Management Review. 2004;**29**:388-403

[27] Evans JR, Dean JW Jr. Total Quality: Management, Organization, and Strategy. 2nd ed. South-Western: Cincinnati, OH; 2000

[28] Shortell SM, O'Brien JL, Carman JM, Foster RW, Hughes EF, Boerstler H, et al. Assessing the impact of continuous quality improvement/total quality management: Concept versus implementation. Health Services Research. 1995;**30**:377

[29] Weil M, Reisch M, Ohmer ML. The Handbook of Community Practice. 2nd ed. Thousand Oaks, CA: Sage Publications, Inc; 2012

[30] Hewison A. Evidence-based medicine: What about evidence-based management? Journal of Nursing Management. 1997;**5**:195-198

[31] Grogan CM, Abraham AJ, Westlake M. Medicaid Managed Care Organizations' Substance Use Disorder Coverage Policies 2016-2017. New Orleans, LA: Academy Health Annual Research Meeting; 2017

[32] Marsh JC, Cao D, Guerrero EG, Shin HC. Need-service matching in substance abuse treatment: Racial/ethnic differences. Evaluation and Program Planning. 2009;**32**:43-51

[33] Andrews CM, Guerrero GE, Wooten NR, Lengnick-Hall R. The Medicaid expansion gap and racial and

ethnic minorities with substance use disorders. American Journal of Public Health. 2015;**105**:S452-S454

[34] Guerrero EG, Garner B, Cook B, Kong Y, Vega W, Gelberg L. Identifying and reducing disparities in successful addiction treatment completion: Testing the role of Medicaid. Substance Abuse Treatment, Prevention, and Policy. 2017;**12**:27

[35] Frimpong JA, D'Aunno T, Jiang L. Determinants of the availability of hepatitis c testing services in opioid treatment programs: Results from a national study. American Journal of Public Health. 2014;**106**:75-82. DOI: 10.2105/AJPH.2013.301827

[36] Frimpong JA, Stewart LM, Singh KP, Rivers PA, Sejong B. Health information technology capacity at federally qualified health centers: A mechanism for improving quality of care. BMC Health Services Research. 2013;**13**:1-12. DOI: 10.1186/1472-6963-13-35

[37] D'Aunno T, Friedmann PD, Chen Q, Wilson DM. Integration of substance abuse treatment organizations into accountable care organizations: Results from a national survey. Journal of Health Politics, Policy and Law. 2015;**40**:797-819

[38] D'Aunno T, Broffman L, Sparer M, Kumar S. Factors that distinguish high- performing accountable care organizations in the medicare shared savings program. Health Services Research. 2016;**53**(1):120-137. DOI: 10.1111/1475-6773.12642

[39] Randall-David E. Strategies for Working with Culturally Diverse Communities and Clients. Washington, DC: Association for the Care of Children's Health; 1989

[40] Howard DL. Culturally competent treatment of African American clients among a national sample of outpatient substance abuse treatment units. Journal of Substance Abuse Treatment. 2003;**24**:89-102

[41] Horvat L, Horey D, Romios P, Kis-Rigo J. Cultural competence education for health professionals. Cochrane Database of Systematic Reviews. 2014;**5**:CD009405. DOI: 10.1002/14651858.CD009405.pub2

[42] Guerrero EG. Managerial capacity and adoption of culturally competent practices in outpatient substance abuse treatment organizations. Journal of Substance Abuse Treatment. 2010;**39**:329-339. DOI: 10.1016/j.jsat.2010.07.004

[43] Gallardo ME, Curry SJ. Shifting perspectives: Culturally responsive interventions with Latino substance abusers. Journal of Ethnicity in Substance Abuse. 2009;**8**:314-329. DOI: 10.1080/15332640903110492

[44] Howard DL. Are the treatment goals of culturally competent outpatient substance abuse treatment units congruent with their client profile? Journal of Substance Abuse Treatment. 2003;**24**:103-113

[45] Campbell CI, Alexander JA. Culturally competent treatment practices and ancillary service use in outpatient substance abuse treatment. Journal of Substance Abuse Treatment. 2002;**22**:109-119

[46] Bowser BP, Bilal R. Drug treatment effectiveness: African-American culture in recovery. Journal of Psychoactive Drugs. 2001;**33**:391-402

[47] Guerrero GE, Andrews C. Cultural competence in outpatient substance abuse treatment: Measurement and relationship with wait time and retention. Drug and Alcohol Dependence. 2011;**119**:e13-e22. DOI: 10.1016/j.drugalcdep.2011.05.020

[48] Katarzyna T, Steinka-Fry EE, Tanner-Smith GA, Dakof CH. Culturally sensitive substance use treatment for racial/ethnic minority youth: A meta-analytic review. Journal of Substance Abuse Treatment. 2017;**75**:22-37

[49] Guerrero GE, Campos M, Urada D, Yang JC. Do cultural and linguistic competence matter in Latinos' completion of mandated substance abuse treatment? Substance Abuse Treatment, Prevention, and Policy. 2012;7:34

[50] Guerrero GE, Henwood B, Wenzel S. Service integration to reduce homelessness in Los Angeles County: Multiple stakeholders' perspective. Human Service Organizations Management. 2014;**38**:44-54. DOI: 10.1080/03643107.2013.853009

[51] Guerrero GE. Organizational characteristics fostering adoption of culturally competent practices in outpatient substance abuse treatment in the U.S. Evaluation and Program Planning. 2012;**35**:9-15. DOI: 10.1016/j.evalprogplan.2011.06.001

[52] Guerrero GE, Kim A. Organizational structure, leadership, and readiness for change and the implementation of organizational cultural competence in addiction health services. Evaluation and Program Planning. 2013;**40**:74-81. DOI: 10.1016/j.evalprogplan.2013.05.0

[53] Guerrero EG, Khachikian T, Kim T, Kong Y, Vega WA. Spanish language proficiency among providers and Latino clients' engagement in substance abuse treatment. Addictive Behaviors. 2013;**38**:2893-2897

[54] Chow J, Austin MJ. The culturally responsive social service agency: The application of an evolving definition to a case study. Administration in Social Work. 2008;**32**(3):39-64

[55] Austin MJ, Regan K, Gothard S, Carnochan S. Becoming a manager in a nonprofit human service organization: Making the transition from specialist to generalist. Administration in Social Work. 2013;**37**(4):372-385

Chapter 6

Leadership Approaches to Developing an Effective Drug Treatment System

Erick G. Guerrero and Tenie Khachikian

Abstract

Improving the effectiveness of the substance use disorder (SUD) treatment requires leadership approaches that have an impact on the effectiveness of drug treatment. To promote this positive system change, we define leadership beyond leaders' characteristics. We consider leadership as a developmental competency among individuals, as well as the relational role of followers and the enabling context of organizational climate which together create a system of influence. Using this developing framework, we discuss how the foundations of certain leadership styles, like transformational leadership can be enacted by program leaders to improve the human and program resources necessary to deliver culturally responsive and evidence-based treatment for some of the most vulnerable groups struggling with SUDs. Building on their transformational and implementation competencies, program leaders can promote organizational climates and program and financial approaches to deliver effective care to some of the most vulnerable populations. We provide a case study to stimulate discussion on how leadership can trickle down to staff to improve care for vulnerable clients.

Keywords: leadership, organizational climate, diversity, evidence-based practice, treatment effectiveness

1. Introduction

Leaders in substance use disorder (SUD) treatment organizations face significant challenges to improve the effectiveness of drug treatment system. Among the most significant challenges are responding to an increasingly diverse client population with high rates of co-occurring medical conditions and high levels of comorbidity [1]. To deliver such practices, program leaders, which represent mainly managers (directors and supervisors) need to have a workforce with reduced rates of burnout and mitigate this and other factors that lead to high turnover rates as well [1–3]. Additionally, program leaders need to prepare the treatment workforce to deliver evidence-based practices and sustain that delivery overtime. To do so, program leaders require leadership to implement practices that are effective and culturally responsive.

SUD treatment programs overall are challenged by limited human and program resources and poorly organized financial incentives and payment systems [4]. Leaders of these programs constantly seek to stabilize funding, improve technical resources, and mitigate the risk of staff turnover [1, 5, 6]. These factors alone handicap program's ability to deliver effective services [4]. Despite these challenges, program administrators have limited formal training to increase the level of readiness of counselors to deliver evidence-based practices and measure client outcomes [2, 3, 7, 8]. SUD treatment leaders face increasing pressures from federal and state institutions to deliver evidence-based practices (EBPs) to reduce disparities between health outcomes of racial and ethnic minorities compared to Whites [9, 10]. Leadership is a key factor associated with implementation of EBPs given that organizational leaders are generally responsible for overseeing the implementation process [11]. It is necessary to understand how leadership can influence the effectiveness of care in SUD treatment.

Transformational leadership is the type of leadership that has the most empirical support in the extant literature [12]. It is generally characterized by the leader's ability to inspire others to follow a particular course of action [13]. These leaders draw from the unique talents of each staff member, provide them feedback based on staff needs, stimulate their problem solving abilities and create a sense of shared purpose [13, 14]. Although transactional leadership, which is based on reinforcing performance using rewards is also commonly used by managers [15–17], transformational leadership has demonstrated a higher impact motivating staff to improve performance, which in behavioral health generally translates into delivering treatment with fidelity [12, 14, 18].

The extant literature suggests that leadership affects implementation of EBPs both directly and indirectly by shaping the organizational context, which then influences employee behaviors [19]. This chapter focused on a deeper understanding of the leaders' relationship with followers and the role of context (organizational climate), in facilitating leadership across the organization. We focus mainly on transformational leadership and the context of service delivery of SUD treatment.

We begin laying the theoretical foundation of ways in which leadership at the director or upper management level may influence treatment staff (supervisors and counselors) to improve care. Then we highlight the differential training necessary for upper and middle level managers to improve the implementation and impact of effective practices. Upper managers need leadership training on creating buy-in using role modeling and promoting employees' professional development. In contrast, middle managers (supervisors) need leadership training on implementation approaches to prioritize, guide, promote and supervise implementation of needed practice to improve the effectiveness of care. Together, leadership at the upper and middle management levels can make a difference in improving the quality of care in SUD treatment systems.

In building a comprehensive framework of leadership in SUD treatment, we consider the role of context (i.e., organizational climate) to support the delivery of EBPs in SUD treatment. Organizational climate is considered employees' shared perception of what is rewarded, promoted, and punished in their organization. Because leaders' communication and prioritization generally show what is rewarded, promoted and punished in the workplace, it is critical to examine the relationship between leadership and climate. For instance, program directors' prioritization of new norms and expectations (e.g., quality of care) may influence counselor's adoption of those norms and endorsement of congruent practices (e.g., EBPs). Because the organizational climate (context) supports and encourages employees in implementing a new practice [20] the leader-climate-practice mechanism is critical to improve the quality of care.

Researchers have explored the leader–climate–practice mechanism in diverse fields, such as industrial safety [21], corporate customer services [22], and evidence-based health care practices [23]. Exploration of the extent to which this mechanism applies to implementing effective practices in SUD treatment is warranted.

To contextualize the leader-climate-practice mechanism in SUD, it is critical to describe the structure of this system. SUD treatment programs in the United States are generally small with an average of five to six employees, with less than 1 million in revenue and with a mix of professional and paraprofessional counselors. That is, the field has a significant number of counselors in recovery with limited formal academic education. Because these programs are small, managers have a frequent and strong relationship with treatment staff. Because the relationship among program staff is close, leadership and climate can be considered major drivers of organizational change.

The following narrative describes the theory and application of two main mechanisms whereby leadership among program directors influence middle managers (i.e. supervisors) and in turn counselors on: (1) how directorial leadership may influence middle managers and direct service staff and (2) how a supportive context, (i.e., organizational climate) may enhance the influence of leadership on direct service staff implementation of effective or EBPs.

2. Leadership across management and direct service staff

2.1 Theoretical framework

Research suggests that director's transformational leadership is necessary to ensure the implementation of policies and practices [24] with limited studies examining the role of middle managers to contribute to implementation [25]. Leadership at different levels of management is one mechanism for implementing needed practices to improve the effectiveness of SUD treatment programs. Because SUD treatment programs generally have a director and supervisor who plays a leadership role in direct change, it is important to distinguish their contribution to improving effectiveness in treatment.

To distinguish the contribution of directors and supervisors' leadership to effectively implement EBPs, we discuss the leadership of both top and middle managers in the implementation process. For instance, how directors' transformational leadership (ability to inspire employees to follow a particular course of action) and middle managers' implementation leadership (supporting staff in implementing EBPs) may support counselors' efforts to deliver EBPs. These EBPs can include the most common and effective practices, such as contingency management treatment (CMT) and medication-assisted treatment (MAT). CMT is a psychosocial intervention based on principles of behavior modification (e.g., clients receive a gift card for a clean drug test) with significant empirical support [26]. MAT is a pharmacological intervention that relies on specific drugs (e.g. buprenorphine, vivitrol, and naloxone) to reduce cravings or block effects for alcohol and illegal drugs. Delivering these two EBPs in SUD treatment would increase its effectiveness. Unfortunately, only one third of programs offer these EBPs in the United States [27], and if offered, they are poorly or inconsistently delivered [28, 29].

2.2 Top managers' transformational leadership

Treatment staff may benefit from transformational leadership from their program directors. That is, directors may communicate values, goals and vision to develop a system to improve decision making. Directors enacting transformational leadership can influence treatment staff attitudes toward, adoption and implementation of, and use of EBPs in SUD treatment [30]. In particular, directors may enhance their energy and attention in promoting staff's professional growth and gaining their trust in director's vision. For example, on the implementation of EBPs, directors may invest in gaining buy-in from middle managers about approaches to improve quality of care, and buy-in from counselors about the benefits of delivering EBPs and achieving recovery results for clients.

2.3 Middle managers' implementation leadership

Whereas program directors may direct their energy in creating buy-in about the benefits of delivering EBPs, middle managers or supervisors can focus on communicating management commitment to implementation of EBPs [31]. Middle managers have different mechanisms to focus on this commitment through communication, training, coaching, and encouragement [32] that lead staff to changing service delivery behaviors [33].

Growing attention on middle managers' abilities to communicate, integrate, interpret, and synthesize issues are critical to support the concrete needs of counselors to implement EBPs [33]. A recently developed framework of implementation leadership is based on the foundation of middle managers' leadership approaches to be (1) proactive, (2) knowledgeable, (3) supportive and (4) perseverant to best support the implementation efforts. (1) Proactive leadership consists of problem solving behavior to accomplish implementation, while (2) knowledge leadership is well connected to the authority of knowledge about an EBP and its implementation needs; (3) Supportive leadership, authors argue is necessary to recognize, appreciate and guide employee' implementation efforts and (4) perseverant leadership challenges leaders to carry through the challenges, and address issues that may cause the implementation to falter. Together, these four categories are connected to leadership literature that is critical in influencing others, but in this case target implementation of EBPs.

When managers consistently communicate the priority of and act to support the implementation of a practice, they are more likely to influence employee action [34]. Communication with employees must come from middle managers who are the proximate manager to guide staff through the concrete, technical and cultural aspects of delivering effective treatment. Moreover, knowledgeable, supportive, and consistent approaches are expected from middle managers as staff engage in the implementation of a novel practice. Top managers or directors in turn, should focus on supporting supervisors and employees in engaging in the implementation and constantly communicate the mission and get buy-in into the overall goal of the program and commitment to quality of care.

Leadership influence across management is a social exchange across individuals with different roles, status, competencies, and responsibilities [35]. Hence, we argue that there is a cascading influence of multilevel leadership, from top managers to middle managers and from middle managers to employee attitudes and behaviors.

It is not clear how managers enacting different leadership styles operate simultaneously to influence front line workers' performance [36]. Some research has explored how specific leadership approaches and organizational context support the implementation of effective practices that improve organizational performance [37]. Although the leader–follower relationship is critical to create and promote organizational change [34], it is not clear how leaders can impact this relationship to achieve desired outcomes. We discussed the critical relationship among three main actors (top manager, middle manager and counselor) in the implementation process, but the enabling context of organizational climate may facilitate or restrict leaders' influence on organizational change.

3. Leadership and organizational climate influence on staff

Defined as employees' shared perception of what is expected, promoted, supported, rewarded and punished within the workplace, organizational climate could be considered a product of leadership. Leaders shape the norms and practices of the workplace, which can directly and indirectly influence implementation practices. This is particularly the case in SUD treatment programs that are generally small, hierarchical, and intimate.

3.1 Theoretical framework

Because transformational leadership behaviors are proven to create organizational change, it is warranted to consider transformational leaders to create an organizational context conducive to implementing new practices. The extant literature suggests that leaders positively or negatively contribute to the creation, development, and sustainment of an organizational climate that fosters employee attitudes and behaviors that support innovative practice use [38–40]. In a strong implementation climate, employees perceive new practices as a priority rather than a distraction or disruption [41, 42]. Several studies have found a positive association between implementation climate and implementation effectiveness, although empirical studies of implementation climate are limited [43–45].

3.2 Organizational climate as a supporting factor in implementation and quality of care

The extant literature suggests that leaders may shape organizational climate through a social learning process in which staff members repeatedly interact with and observe their leader to interpret organizational priorities [39, 46]. In their interaction with followers, leaders communicate the importance of various tasks through their behavior and interactions with employees. In SUD treatment, leaders develop strategic goals to communicate their organizational mission, monitor and supervise staff activities, model desired behavior, and reward staff behavior in line with the prioritized behavior or outcome [47–49].

Experts suggest that leaders rely on three main approaches to communicate priorities They explicitly or implicitly communicate what behavior or attitudes they value, what behavior or attitudes should be rewarded, what behavior or attitudes should be punished. By communicating their expectations and priorities in these ways, leaders develop, support, and perpetuate an organizational climate [50].

4. Ethnic leaders' influence on the implementation of cultural competence

The cultural background of individuals with decision making power and leadership potential has also become an important factor to consider in the study of long-term implementation of culturally responsive practices [51]. Managers' ethnic background may enhance their commitment to cultural practices that represent their values and experiences serving racial/ethnic minorities. This familiarity with cultural background and life experience may be a powerful enabler of implementation of culturally responsive and evidence-based practices. There is a need to address implementation in this context, as it can help SUD treatment programs located in minority communities to consistently respond to the cultural and language service needs of racial and ethnic minority patients [52].

We propose that it is critical to explore how leadership cascades from top management to direct service, how climate can be an enabling factor to deliver quality of care, and finally how the ethnic background of transformational leaders may help the implementation process that included service practices that are culturally tailored, and directed toward cultural minorities.

Although there may be other barriers and facilitators of implementation of culturally responsive and evidence-based practices, as well as an abundant literature on leadership approaches to promote organizational change, this chapter describes active components of leadership and the organizational context that may drive the implementation of EBPs in SUD treatment organizations. By enacting leadership styles at different levels, and promoting a supporting climate for implementation, SUD treatment leaders may work on specific transformational behaviors among directors, implementation leadership at the supervisor level, and organizational climate to support the implementation process.

Although the characteristics of leaders are associated with organizational outcomes, critical characteristics like ethnic background is associated with increased commitment to deliver culturally responsive SUD treatment. Ethnic minority leaders may enhance the delivery of quality of care in SUD treatment to minority clients.

5. Implications for management to support treatment effectiveness

The proposed conceptual model highlights how leadership, conceptualized as influence on employees to deliver quality of care relies on managers at different levels, and can be supported by the climate of the organization. Because individuals within SUD treatment programs have different roles, responsibilities and skills, it is important to understand how each of these individuals may best prepare to implement culturally responsive and evidence-based care that enhance treatment effectiveness.

Upper managers, or program directors should consider building on their leadership abilities to communicate a vision for the treatment programs consistent with treatment effectiveness. Directors should also build competencies to appraise individual strengths, communicate them to staff, and learn how to link these strengths with program goals. To accomplish this task, directors should allow themselves to spend significant time and resources positively relating to staff, including middle managers or supervisors. Obtaining buy-in from supervisors should be one of the director's goal. By developing credibility and trust among supervisors, directors would be able to reach direct service staff, or counselors. In short, directors should invest in transformational leadership qualities that build on a genuine person with a clear view of what is to be accomplished and with a sincere approach to supporting the professional growth of staff.

Middle managers or [clinical] supervisors should consider building on their leadership abilities to help staff effectively implement practices. Building on capacities to be proactive and respond to staff questions and comments about the implementation process or the practice to be implemented is critical. Supervisors should also invest in developing the knowledge of both the implementation process as well as the EBPs considered for implementation and ways to evaluate their outcomes. Supervisors should also demonstrate supportive leadership to recognize, appreciate, and guide staff's implementation efforts. Finally, the supervisor's need to role model perseverant leadership to carry through the challenges and address all the many shortcomings during the implementation process. These four approaches provide a capacity-building plan for supervisors to enhance the transformational leadership efforts from their program directors, and contribute concrete capacities to influencing staff to deliver quality of care.

Both, upper and middle managers, using their own leadership approach can start shaping the organizational climate of the treatment organization. But for the climate to be a driver of quality of care, both manager types need to be consistent in communicating their priorities to treatment staff and reducing any contingencies that may keep staff from achieving program goals. Supplementing an organizational climate that supports the delivery of culturally responsive and evidence-based care can become an active driver of quality of care.

6. Case example

John Clark, a Caucasian male in his upper 60s was generally regarded as a friendly and hard-working program director. He managed one of over 400 substance use disorder treatment programs located in one of the largest cities in the West Coast. Like most others, his program had a supervisor overseeing 5 counselors, 3 coordinators and 2 office staff. Mr. Clark was often proud that he promoted a great sense of collegiality among his staff and that his workplace was always jovial and productive. During state and county meetings, he also reaffirmed his commitment to cultural competence in response to the increasing client diversity in his program. Almost half of his clients were women, and 70 percent self-report a non-White racial background.

During program meetings, Mr. Clark emphasized the importance of delivering evidence-based practices tailored to their diverse population. He often delivered expectations with a great sense of humor, which made program meetings entertaining. But staff were growing frustrated by the lack of meaningful support to implement the proposed EBPs. Staff were also constantly confused how to adapt EBPs to meet the service needs of women, Latinos and African Americans, their main demographics.

Among his peers at other programs, Mr. Clark was a leader in the field, while in his program, there was an increasing frustration by what many saw as "empty rhetoric." Meanwhile, Ms. Jenkins, a 55-year-old Caucasian clinical supervisor spent most of her time dealing with billing and human resources issues, not able to provide meaningful support to deliver quality of care. Treatment staff were constantly pulled in different directions to comply with billing issues, while their professional development and self-efficacy needs were not addressed.

Juan Lopez, a 60-year-old Latino counselor was the most vocal staff complaining about the lack of counselor diversity and limited evaluation of program effectiveness. For years, he had requested additional Spanish speaking counselors with training in mental health issues to respond to the increasing numbers of Latino clients suffering from mental health and substance use disorders. Juan and some of his peer also needed more training to respond to the higher severity of mental health issues they were encountering with their clients. The treatment staff requested more guidance and evaluation of their current practices. They grew frustrated with an increasing number of clients who passed through their program two to three times a year with limited signs of progress.

These program and service delivery concerns started to reach funders and Mr. Clark's leadership on delivering effective and culturally responsive care was being challenged among his peers. The program was losing funding. Some funders suspended funding or added restrictions based on showing evidence of program performance. Two of the five treatment staff and one of the office staff resigned and move to another nearby program.

1. Why would programs falter with Mr. Clark's kind of leadership?

2. How does his leadership trickle down to his supervisor and staff?

3. What did Mr. Clark, as program director need to do to ensure his treatment staff was prepared to deliver culturally responsive and evidence-based care?

4. What did Mr. Clark, as a leader need to do to ensure his treatment staff was prepared to deliver culturally responsive and evidence-based care?

5. To what extent Mr. Clark would benefit from developing competencies in transformational leadership?

6. To what extent Ms. Jenkins would benefit from developing competencies in implementation leadership?

7. What may be key approaches to developing a competent and diverse treatment workforce?

7. Conclusion

Leaders in SUD treatment face significant challenges to improve the effectiveness of drug treatment. As this treatment system must withstand funding uncertainty, limited technical resources and workforce development needs [1, 5, 6], program managers require unique leadership approaches. Training managers to develop their leadership capacity to help their staff implement EBPs with fidelity has become a unique feature to improve effectiveness needs in this system [53].

However, like other human service organizations, program leaders in SUD treatment may need to develop a comprehensive organizational development plan. This plan may include a professional pipeline to prepare counselors and early managers from racial and ethnic minority backgrounds to become competent middle and upper managers [54]. This approach would response to the increasing cultural diversity in the client population, as well as the diversity of their co-occurring medical conditions.

The framework proposed in this chapter highlights some of the most significant problems that the SUD treatment system faces—funding, technology and workforce. We discussed a leadership approach that assumes a trickledown effect where leading managers are more likely to develop effective counselors, and where these counselors are better prepared to respond to the recovery service needs of a diverse client population.

To enhance and sustain effectiveness in SUD treatment, a leadership capacity plan may also include a succession planning and alignment. Leaders in the SUD treatment system may reduce uncertainty in operations and funding and increase equity and inclusion with a comprehensive vision. The extant literature on leadership offers a wealth of examples on how leaders' vision activates followers and lead to organizational effectiveness [12–14].

To support the delivery of effective care, competent leaders may promote an organizational climate of trust and align resources to sustain service delivery [54]. This organizational climate can enable learning among staff to gradually improve the quality of care. Moreover, having an effective and inclusive succession plan and a climate of trust and support may become the driver of quality of care. In short, it may be that through the development of transformational leadership that program managers may be able to shape the human and program resources to reliably help clients achieve recovery.

To help SUD treatment systems to deliver effective care, a research agenda needs to consider modifiable organizational factors that make evidence-based treatment effective. One of these drivers is leadership, considered "influence" in the system. Organizational interventions need to include leaders, followers and context to have a "system of influence" that impact effectiveness. Policy makers, healthcare administrators, program managers and counselors may benefit from developing this leadership approach to improve recovery.

Acknowledgements

We would like to acknowledge the support and contributions of the Integrated Substance Abuse Treatment to Eliminate Disparities (www.isated.com) research team. In particular, we recognize the support of Veronica Serret, Angelique Montgomery and Yinfei Kong to develop the material presented in this chapter. We would also like to acknowledge the support and feedback provided by the Los Angeles County Department of Public Health leaders and in particular, Dr. Tina Kim, the director of research for the Substance Abuse Prevention and Control.

Conflict of interest

The authors declare no conflict of interest.

Thanks

We thank the large network of treatment providers that have provided feedback to different versions of the material presented in this chapter through their participation in the numerous research projects conducted in Los Angeles County, California. Without their support and feedback, the authors could not have developed the material presented in this chapter.

Abbreviations

CMT	contingency management treatment
MAT	medication-assisted treatment
EBPs	evidence-based practices
SUD	substance use disorder

Author details

Erick G. Guerrero[1*] and Tenie Khachikian[2]

1 I-Lead Institute, Research to End Healthcare Disparities Corp, Santa Monica, CA, United States

2 University of Chicago, Chicago, IL, United States

*Address all correspondence to: erickguerrero454@gmail.com

References

[1] Substance Abuse and Mental Health Services Administration. Substance abuse treatment facilities provide programs to fit clients; 2007. Available from: http://www.samhsa.gov/newsroom/advisories/0706140319.aspx

[2] Center for Substance Abuse Treatment (CSAT). Clinical supervision and professional development of the substance abuse counselor. Treatment Improvement Protocol (TIP) Series 52, DHHS Publication No. (SMA) 09-4377. Rockville, MD: Substance Abuse and Mental Health Administration; 2009a

[3] Center for Substance Abuse Treatment (CSAT). Implementing change in substance abuse treatment programs. Treatment Improvement Protocol (TIP) Series 31, DHHS Publication No. (SMA) 09-4377. Rockville, MD: Substance Abuse and Mental Health Administration; 2009b

[4] McLellan AT, Carise D, Kleber HD. Can the national addiction treatment infrastructure support the public's demand for quality care? Journal of Substance Abuse Treatment. 2003;**25**(2):117-121. DOI: 10.1016/S0740-5472(03)00156-9

[5] D'Aunno T. The role of organization and management in substance abuse treatment: Review and roadmap. Journal of Substance Abuse Treatment. 2006;**31**:221-233

[6] Roman PM, Ducharme LJ, Knudsen HK. Patterns of organization and management in private and public substance abuse treatment programs. Journal of Substance Abuse Treatment. 2006;**31**(3):235-243. DOI: 10.1016/j.jsat.2006.06.017

[7] Fixsen DL, Naoom SF, Blase KA, Friedman RM, Wallace F. Implementation research: A synthesis of the literature. FMHI Publication No. 231. Tampa, FL: University of South Florida, Louis de la Parte Florida Mental Health Institute, National Implementation Research Network; 2005

[8] Rawson R, McCleland T. Healthcare reform and treatment: Changes in organization, financing, and standards of care. Posted presented at the meeting of County Alcohol and Drug Program Administrators' Association of California. Sacramento, California; 2010

[9] Institute of Medicine. Crossing the Quality Chasm: A New Health System for the Twenty-First Century. Washington, DC: National Academies Press; 2001

[10] Institute of Medicine. Unequal Treatment: Confronting Racial and Ethnic Disparities in Health Care. Washington, DC: National Academies Press; 2013

[11] Battilana J, Gilmartin M, Sengul M, Pache AC, Alexander JA. Leadership competencies for implementing planned organizational change. The Leadership Quarterly. 2010;**21**:422-438

[12] Judge TA, Piccolo RF. Transformational and transactional leadership: A meta-analytic test of their relative validity. The Journal of Applied Psychology. 2004;**89**:755-768

[13] Bass BM, Avolio BJ. Improving Organizational Effectiveness through Transformational Leadership. Thousand Oaks: Sage; 1994

[14] Bass BM, Avolio BJ, Jung DI, Berson Y. Predicting unit performance by assessing transformational and transactional leadership. The Journal of Applied Psychology. 2003;**88**:207-218

[15] Aarons GA, Ehrhart MG, Farahnak LR, Sklar M. Aligning

leadership across systems and organizations to develop a strategic climate for evidence-based. Annual Review of Public Health. 2014;**35**:255-274

[16] Aarons GA, Ehrhart MG, Moullin JC, Torres EM, Green AE. Testing the leadership and organizational change for implementation (LOCI) intervention in substance abuse treatment: A cluster randomized trial study protocol. Implementation Science. 2016;**12**(1):29

[17] Aarons GA, Ehrhart MG, Farahnak LR. The implementation leadership scale (ILS): Development of a brief measure of unit level implementation leadership. Implementation Science. 2014;**9**:45

[18] Aarons GA. Transformational and transactional leadership: Association with attitudes toward evidence-based practice. Psychiatric Services. 2006;**57**:1162-1169. DOI: 10.1176/appi.ps.57.8.1162

[19] Dinh JE, Lord RG, Gardner WL, Meuser JD, Liden RC, Hu J. Leadership theory and research in the new millennium: Current theoretical trends and changing perspectives. The Leadership Quarterly. 2014;**25**:36-62

[20] Zohar D. The effects of leadership dimensions, safety climate, and assigned priorities on minor injuries in work groups. Journal of Organizational Behavior. 2002;**23**:75-92

[21] Zohar D. Safety climate: Conceptualization, measurement, and improvement. In: Schneider B, Barbera KM, editors. The Oxford Handbook of Organizational Climate and Culture. New York: Oxford University Press; 2014. pp. 317-334

[22] Schneider B, Ehrhart MG, Macey WH. Organizational climate and culture. Annual Review of Psychology. 2013;**64**:361-388

[23] Aarons GA, Ehrhart MG, Farahnak LR, Sklar M. Aligning leadership across systems and organizations to develop strategic climate for evidence-based practice implementation. Annual Review of Public Health. 2014;**35**:255-274

[24] Guerrero GE, Kim A. Organizational structure, leadership and readiness for change and the implementation of organizational cultural competence in addiction health services. Evaluation and Program Planning. 2013;**40**:74-81

[25] Aarons GA, Ehrhart MG, Farahnak LR, Hurlburt MS. Leadership and organizational change for implementation (LOCI): A randomized mixed method pilot study of a leadership and organization development intervention for evidence-based practice implementation. Implementation Science. 2015;**10**:11

[26] Prendergast M, Podus D, Finney J, Greenwell L, Roll J. Contingency management for treatment of substance use disorders: A meta-analysis. Addiction. 2006;**101**:1546-1560. DOI: 10.1111/j.1360-0443.2006.01581.x

[27] Knudsen HK, Abraham AJ, Oser CB. Barriers to the implementation of medication-assisted treatment for substance use disorders: The importance of funding policies and medical infrastructure. Evaluation and Program Planning. 2011;**34**:375-381. DOI: 10.1016/j.evalprogplan.2011.02.004

[28] Manuel JK, Hagedorn HJ, Finney JW. Implementing evidence-based psychosocial treatment in specialty substance use disorder care. Psychology of Addictive Behaviors. 2011;**25**:225

[29] McGovern MP, Carroll KM. Evidence-based practices for substance use disorders. The Psychiatric Clinics of North America. 2003;**26**:991

[30] Guerrero EG, Padwa H, Fenwick K, Harris LM, Aarons GA. Identifying and ranking implicit leadership strategies to promote evidence-based practice implementation in addiction health services. Implementation Science. 2016;**11**:69. DOI: 10.1186/s13012-016-0438-y

[31] Birken SA, Lee SYD, Weiner BJ, Chin MH, Chiu M, Schaefer CT. From strategy to action: How top managers' support increases middle managers' commitment to innovation implementation in healthcare organizations. Health Care Management Review. 2015;**40**:159

[32] Engle RL, Lopez ER, Gormley KE, Chan JA, Charns MP, Lukas CV. What roles do middle managers play in implementation of innovative practices? Health Care Management Review. 2016;**42**:14-27

[33] Birken SA, Lee SY, Weiner BJ. Uncovering middle managers' role in healthcare innovation implementation. Implementation Science. 2012;**2**(27):28

[34] Schein EH, Schein P. Organizational Culture and Leadership. 5th ed. San Francisco: Jossey-Bass; 2017

[35] Gottfredson RK, Aguinis H. Leadership behaviors and follower performance: Deductive and inductive examination of theoretical rationales and underlying mechanisms. Journal of Organizational Behavior. 2017;**38**: 558-591. DOI: 10.1002/job.2152

[36] Avolio BJ, Gardner WL, Walumbwa FO, Luthans F, May DR. Unlocking the mask: A look at the process by which authentic leaders impact follower attitudes and behaviors. The Leadership Quarterly. 2004;**15**:801-823

[37] Saboe KN, Taing MU, Way JD, Johnson RE. Examining the unique mediators that underlie the effects of different dimensions of transformational leadership. Journal of Leadership & Organizational Studies. 2015;**22**:175-186. DOI: 10.1177/1548051814561028

[38] Aarons GA, Sommerfeld DH. Leadership, innovation climate, and attitudes toward evidence-based practice during a statewide implementation. Journal of the American Academy of Child and Adolescent Psychiatry. 2012;**51**:423-431

[39] Dragoni L. Understanding the emergence of state goal orientation in organizational work groups: The role of leadership and multilevel climate perceptions. The Journal of Applied Psychology. 2005;**90**:1084-1095

[40] Michaelis B, Stegmaier R, Sonntag K. Shedding light on followers' innovation implementation behavior: The role of transformational leadership, commitment to change, and climate for initiative. Journal of Managerial Psychology. 2010;**25**:408-429

[41] Klein KJ, Sorra JS. The challenge of innovation implementation. The Academy of Management Review. 1996;**21**:1055-1080

[42] Klein KJ, Knight AP. Innovation implementation: Overcoming the challenge. Current Directions in Psychological Science. 2005;**14**:243-246

[43] Klein KJ, Conn AB, Sorra JS. Implementing computerized technology: An organizational analysis. The Journal of Applied Psychology. 2001;**86**:811-824

[44] Holahan PJ, Aronson ZH, Jurkat MP, Schoorman FD. Implementing computer

technology: A multiorganizational test of Klein and Sorra's model. Journal of Engineering and Technology Management. 2004;**21**:31-50

[45] Dong L, Neufeld DJ, Higgins C. Testing Klein and Sorra's innovation implementation model: An empirical examination. Journal of Engineering and Technology Management. 2008;**25**:237-255

[46] Bandura A. Social Foundations of Thought and Action: A Social-Cognitive View. Englewood Cliffs: Prentice-Hall; 1986

[47] Schein EA. Organizational Culture and Leadership. 2nd ed. San Francisco: Jossey-Bass; 1992

[48] Wimbush JC, Shepard JM. Toward an understanding of ethical climate: Its relationship to ethical behavior and supervisory influence. Journal of Business Ethics. 1994;**13**:637-647

[49] Zohar D. The influence of leadership and climate on occupational health and safety. In: Hofmann DA, Tetrick LE, editors. Health and Safety in Organizations: A Multilevel Perspective. San Francisco: Jossey-Bass; 2003. pp. 201-230

[50] Zohar D, Luria G. Climate as a social-cognitive construction of supervisory safety practices: Scripts as proxy of behavior patterns. The Journal of Applied Psychology. 2004;**89**:322-333

[51] Guerrero EG, Khachikian T. Frimpoing JA, Howard LD, Kong Y, Hunter S. Drivers of continued implementation of cultural competence in substance use disorder treatment. Journal of Substance Abuse Treatment. 2019;**105**:5-11. DOI: 10.1016/j.jsat.2019.07.009

[52] Delphin-Rittmon M, Andres-Hyman R, Flanagan EH, Ortiz J, Amer MM, Davidson L. Racial-ethnic differences in referral source, diagnosis, and length of stay in inpatient substance abuse treatment. Psychiatric Services. 2012;**63**:612-615

[53] Proctor E, Ramsey AT, Brown MT, et al. Training in implementation practice leadership (TRIPLE): Evaluation of a novel practice change strategy in behavioral health organizations. Implementation Science. 2019;**14**:66. DOI: 10.1186/s13012-019-0906-2

[54] Gothard S, Austin MJ. Leadership succession planning: Implications for nonprofit human service organizations. Administration in Social Work. 2013;**37**(3):272-285. DOI: 10.1080/03643107.2012.684741